CW00369472

MARTIN HIBBERT is a dad of
Martin and his daughter, Eve,
injuries as a result of the Manch
2017. They were the closest people to the bomber to survive. After two separate courses of radical NeuroPhysics Therapy (NPT) in Australia, Martin, who had been left paralysed from the belly button down, regained movement in his legs and was able to stand in his callipers. He is the vice chairman of the Spinal Injuries Association and is also involved in seeking justice for those affected by the Manchester Arena bombing. He hopes to build an NPT clinic in Manchester so all spinal-cord injury patients can receive the same radical treatment. He lives in Chorley with his wife, Gabby, and cocker spaniel, Alfie.

FIONA DUFFY has worked as a journalist for more than thirty years. After graduating from the College of Ripon and York St John with a 2:1 honours degree in English literature and history she became an apprentice journalist with Westminster Press, gaining a diploma in journalism. After seven years working on local newspapers, Fiona moved to women's magazines and, eventually, became a freelance writer for national publications. Her work with victims of crime over two decades has also seen her co-launch and run the high-profile campaign for Helen's Law which was added to the statute book in January 2021. As a result, convicted killers who refuse to disclose the whereabouts of their victims will face longer sentences. Fiona has won two awards for this work: Campaign of the Year 2019 at the British Journalism Awards and the national Making a Difference campaign 2020 for Journalism Matters. Fiona lives in Sutton Coldfield, West Midlands, with her husband, two children and a Sprollie (a springer spaniel-collie cross) dog, Maddie.

Also by Fiona Duffy

Justice for Helen, Marie McCourt with Fiona Duffy

TOP OF THE WORLD

Surviving the Manchester Bombing to Scale Kilimanjaro in a Wheelchair

Martin Hibbert, with Fiona Duffy

G:

First published in the UK in 2024 by Gemini Adult Books Ltd,
part of the Gemini Books Group

Based in Woodbridge and London

Marine House, Tide Mill Way,
Woodbridge, Suffolk IP12 1AP

www.geminibooks.com

Paperback ISBN 9781802471748
eBook ISBN 9781802472370

A CIP catalogue record for this book is available
from the British Library.

Printed in the UK
10 9 8 7 6 5 4 3 2 1

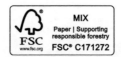

MIX
Paper | Supporting
responsible forestry
FSC® C171272
FSC
www.fsc.org

To my wonderful Mum, Janice
My beautiful daughter, Eve
My soulmate, Gabby

FOREWORD

I'll keep this brief... just read this book but be careful... The resulting inspiration may just change your perspective on everything.

Martin Hibbert is a pretty amazing man. You don't have to spend much time in his company to realise that his passion and enthusiasm can convince anyone to do virtually anything. I haven't often seen him without a smile on his face but, as you would expect for someone who has been through what he has been through, he does have dark days.

In this book he carefully walks you through that darkness but he is always moving towards the light. There are understandable flashbacks to that night at the Manchester Arena and the time spent in hospital. There is the lingering spectre of PTSD. He has to keep busy. He always wants something to look forward to so that he doesn't have to look back.

I don't know about you but Martin is one of those people who makes me think about how I would act if I was in the situation he has found himself in. I wonder if I would be able to think as quickly as he did on the night itself. I wonder how I would react to being told I would never be able to walk again. And I wonder whether I would devote myself to helping others when my own life remains an uphill struggle every single day. I'm pretty sure I wouldn't ever think about climbing a mountain. I still can't quite believe he did it.

His remarkable story has given him a voice and, as you will discover as you read these pages, he knows how to use it. The terrorist at the arena nearly took his life away. He did take the use of his legs away but in spite of that, Martin found that he had also made him stronger than ever.

Martin's real gift is that he is a campaigner. He doesn't make you feel guilty for not doing or supporting something but he convinces you that things need to change by using the sheer weight of reason and sharing his amazing spirit of enthusiasm. It's hard to disagree with that, particularly when you consider the path he has taken to get to where he is. Martin doesn't wear slogan T-shirts but, if he did, his shirt would read 'Don't Write Me Off Because I'm In A Wheelchair'. I don't think there is any danger of that happening.

It has been a real privilege to get to know him over the last few years and to watch his magic at close quarters. I love spending time with him. He makes you look at things in differing ways. He allows you to see things from a new perspective and his motive always seems to be to improve the lives of those around him.

This book is incredible and I hope you love reading it. By the end of it I am sure you will have no doubt in your mind that Martin will go on to achieve great things in life and, if his daughter, Eve, is anything like him, she will too.

Dan Walker

CONTENTS

	Foreword	vii
1.	Little 'Fokker'	1
2.	A Grafter	15
3.	Highs and Increasing Lows	25
4.	Hitting Rock Bottom	37
5.	22 May 2017	47
6.	The Aftermath	60
7.	You'll Never Walk Again	73
8.	The Long Road to Recovery	85
9.	Bowels, Bladders and Breakouts	98
10.	A Whole New World	115
11.	A Miracle Down Under	128
12.	Standing Tall	138
13.	Read All About It	149
14.	A Growing Anger	167
15.	Fighting Back	182
16.	A Bonkers Idea	194
17.	On Top of the World	215

CONTENTS

18. I'm Vindicated… and Trolled   228
19. Dream Believe Achieve   240
    Acknowledgements   251

1

Little 'Fokker'

I'm crouched behind a parked car, as still as a statue. My heart is beating out of my chest.

Seconds creep by.

'I know you're there...' he calls, finally.

Gulp.

'...And I know where you live,' he continues. A prickle of fear runs down my spine and my bladder quivers, threatening to release its contents all over the dusty road. 'Your parents will be hearing about this, you mark my words.'

I remain, hunkered down, long after he gives up and shuffles away, muttering under his breath. Only when my legs start to fizz with pins and needles do I make my move. Summoning my inner Spider-Man powers I scuttle to the next parked car, then the next, before darting up a nearby ginnel.

Phew, I think, leaning back against the red brick wall. Like magic, kids emerge from behind their own hiding places of cars and dustbins and swarm round me. 'Woah, that was close, Hibbert!' they exclaim. Then comes the all-important question. 'What did ya get?' Beady eyes watch, transfixed, as I unfurl my hot fingers to reveal my booty – a tube of Toffo sweets! *Result!* A grin spreads across my face at the reaction – eyes widening in undisguised envy and cries of, 'No way!'

The fear that consumed me just minutes ago has evaporated into the hot summer air. Swaggering now, I tear the paper and chomp my way through each artificially flavoured toffee (no doubt, tossing the wrappers to the ground), steadfastly ignoring the pleas of 'Oh, come on, Hibbert, give us one.'

'Get yer own,' I tell them through a claggy mouthful of strawberry, chocolate and banana sweetness. Recalling this early memory from my childhood makes me realise two things. One – it's little wonder I ended up having so many fillings. (My insatiable sweet tooth has only grown stronger with age.) And, two, the shopkeeper was right. I was a little bugger. Or, to be even more accurate, a little shit. When it came to nicking sweets, the Artful Dodger had nothing on me. I was renowned for my light-fingered prowess at the corner shop on Tonge Moor Road, in Bolton, a few doors down from where we lived.

I'd wait until there was a lull in customers before crawling stealthily through the open door. Pausing near the boxes of crisps, I'd bite my lip in concentration, then slowly, steadily, raise one hand up, up, up towards the sweet counter above. It's like that daring scene involving Tom Cruise in *Mission Impossible* – only far trickier as Tom could actually see what he was doing. I relied on guesswork. Intuition. And luck. Reaching the cool, Perspex counter barrier, I'd snake my hand over the top, then open out my hovering fingers and lower them until they brushed a cellophane wrapper. Knowing that even the tiniest crinkle would give me away, I'd work painstakingly slowly... easing the snaffled item from its resting place. *Come to Martin.* Clasping the contraband, tightly, I'd shuffle backwards through the open door praying I didn't reverse into an unsuspecting old dear. Once outdoors, I'd spring to my feet, then sprint around the corner, into the rear back alley, as fast as my five-year-old legs would carry me.

A Finger of Fudge or packet of Opal Fruits was like winning the jackpot. Fruit Polo sweets were a close second. Mints and Lockets cough sweets were a huge disappointment and gladly distributed

2

to clamouring kids. And Fisherman's Friend lozenges still make me shudder.

It was all great fun until the day the shopkeeper looked up from his newspaper crossword to see a small, grasping hand hovering, like an amusement arcade's claw machine, over his prized confectionery display. By the time he'd thundered 'Oi! – you little...', clambered down off the stool and chased me into the back alley I was long hidden – along with all the kids who'd gathered to watch my latest daring mission. I have no memory of what happened after that near-miss. I like to think I returned to the shop, sticky-mouthed and contrite, promising to change my ways and begging him not to tell on me. Or maybe he did tell – and I've made a mental block of the fireworks that would have, no doubt, resulted (believe me, I'm not exaggerating). Or perhaps he shouted similar threats at all the little scallies pilfering his stock and never followed through.

I smiled at the recent story of how actor Dwayne the 'Rock' Johnson spent almost three hundred dollars buying up every Snickers bar in a 7–Eleven store – to make up for all the ones he'd swiped as a teenager when he was 'broke as hell'. I immediately wanted to copy the gesture. Alas, I was too late. The corner shop has long gone. Mad Betty's Kitchen – a bustling café – now stands in its place. I still feel a guilty pang every time I drive past but, back then, of course, I couldn't see anything wrong with my actions. Money was tight. We couldn't afford sweets. So, I nicked them. It was that simple. I'm such a model citizen these days that people might be surprised at my early childhood and just what a thieving little bugger I was. But it's all part of the person I am today.

As both a proud Boltonian and passionate Greater Mancunian, I won't hear a word said against either my home town or city.

I still get a buzz driving from Chorley to Bolton – coming over the brow of the hill and seeing the dramatic city landscape of Manchester unfurl on my right. It really is the best place in the world to live. But I think it's safe to say that back in the early '80s,

Tonge Moor wasn't top of the list of desirable places. It was all Mum and Dad – newlyweds and new parents – could afford. Back in the '70s, couples settled down and had families young and they were no exception. She and Dad had met on a night out at either the local pub or Conservative club: it would have been one or the other. When it came to courting, no one ventured beyond those parameters.

Mum married at twenty-three and I came along when she was twenty-five. Unlike many other young mums, she juggled motherhood with full-time work in a chemist shop. She really was a trailblazer and I have nothing but admiration for her. I'd see both her and Dad (a policeman) grafting all hours to make ends meet and, once I'd shed my thieving ways, I followed their example.

British summers have become increasingly warm. But, in the Hibbert family, no summer will ever be as hot as the iconic heatwave of 1976 when I made my appearance at Bolton Royal Infirmary on 11 July. We learned never to make a remark about warm weather in Mum's earshot. 'Hot? You think this is hot?' she'd exclaim. Eyes would roll and groans of frustration erupt as she embarked on her all-time favourite story. 'Now, the summer I had Martin, *that* was hot,' she'd begin. 'Out here, I was,' she'd continue, stretching her arms out in front of her for dramatic effect, 'like a bloody elephant. And it were seventy-five degrees. *Seventy-five degrees!* For weeks on end. And we had no air con back then, remember...'

Not only was there no air con, there was no water. With supplies turned off, standpipes were erected in the street. Neighbours, clasping empty buckets, formed orderly queues. Roads melted, train lines buckled, wildfires burned. Britain had never experienced anything like it. I love the fact I was born during such an infamous summer.

It was a difficult birth by all accounts. Not only did I emerge arse first but the cord was wrapped around my neck and I ended up in the special care baby unit for a few days.

Performing the heartbreaking task of clearing out her things with my two younger brothers, we found the commemorative plates she'd proudly had made for each of our births. Mine said '7 lbs' – on the dot. She'd also kept the hospital wrist tags we'd worn as newborns.

From what I remember Mum telling me, I was a good baby and no trouble at all. We lived in a two-up two-down, terraced house on a main road with no front garden. She regularly left me 'getting fresh air' in the pram outside the front door while she got on with the washing. You wouldn't leave your dog tied up outside your front door these days and expect it to still be there two minutes later, but that's what everyone did back then. My earliest memory is of waking up, alone, in a strange room and wondering where me mum was. Climbing out of bed, I padded out of the door and went off looking for her… along a corridor, down an ornate flight of stairs and towards the bright, flashing lights.

And there she was – throwing shapes on the dance floor. I've no idea what the song was but 'Y.M.C.A.' and 'Le Freak' were big back then so it would have been something disco-y. Her lovely smile quickly vanished when she caught sight of me in just my underpants, solemnly sucking a dummy and clutching my blankie. 'Martin!' she screeched, grinding to a halt. 'What are you doing out of bed?' We were on a family holiday at a hotel in the Isle of Man. Within seconds, I'd been scooped up and carted unceremoniously off to bed so my parents could continue their night out. As I said, things were different back then.

I've got two younger brothers but you can forget those heartwarming stories of toddlers adoring new siblings. When Danny came along, in October 1979, I was consumed by jealousy. I vividly remember being taken to the toy shop to choose a toy for the new arrival. I picked out a gleaming Formula 1 toy car that I had no intention of ever handing over. I clutched it tightly to my chest as I peered, unimpressed, at this wailing newborn in my mum's arms and stubbornly thought, *You're* not having it.

Things escalated when he came home. Furious at the fuss everyone was making over this noisy new baby, I went on hunger strike. Days passed and I stubbornly refused to eat a morsel. 'As long as he's drinking, he'll be fine,' doctors assured my frantic parents. There's a photo of me, standing behind Danny in his baby seat, refusing to smile for the camera. There are dark shadows under my eyes and I look pale and wan. After ten days of worrying herself sick, Mum found me in the kitchen with my hand in the biscuit barrel – shovelling the contents into my gob. She never said a word – just tiptoed out again, relieved that I'd finally cracked. But even now, if I'm worried or have a lot on my mind, I can't eat. And that stubbornness has never left me.

With both parents juggling work and a new baby, I was often left to my own devices. When not at school, every single child 'played out'. Holidays and weekends were a continual paradise of non-stop adventures and fun. A typical day involved messing about on the railway track that ran behind our house, endless games of hide-and-seek or tig (catch) in the warren of ginnels and alleys that criss-crossed the estates, lobbing apples and water bombs at windows, making prank calls from public phone boxes and playing knock and run.

I was stopped by the police a few times as, dirty and exhausted, I finally headed home for tea. 'Empty out your pockets,' they'd bark. I never produced anything more than a few old sweet wrappers (having long scoffed the contents). 'Go on, get off home,' they'd order. I never got into real trouble. But I have no doubt that had we stayed there, my life would have turned out very differently. It's one of the reasons Mum and Dad worked such long hours – so they could afford to move. But those early years, getting up to all sorts of mischief, standing my ground against much bigger boys, forging the fiercest of friendships, made me the man I am today. From very early on, I learned to develop a tough outer shell and what some may no doubt call an air of cockiness. That mask of swaggering bravado was adopted and worn no matter how scared I might have been inside. As a result, I've never been bullied and have always been able to stand my corner. Part of it may have been down to my beloved superheroes. I lived and breathed characters like Hulk, Spider-Man and, my absolute favourite, Superman – wearing their T-shirts until they were threadbare and faded. Even at forty-six, I'm still a huge Marvel fan.

We had no car back then so had to walk an hour's journey to school and back along the length of Tonge Moor Road. I remember feeling mutinous at our lack of wheels. I didn't want to be getting splashed by passing cars. I wanted to be inside one. A nice one. Those early years formed a lifelong obsession with motors – and a determination to have a cool car when I grew up. Brollies and waterproofs were for posh kids. If it rained you got wet and stayed in damp, steaming clothes all day. Talking of which, one of my most vivid early memories is of wetting my pants in assembly. I can see myself obediently sitting cross-legged, and watching, with a mixture of fascination and shame, this puddle growing around me on the polished, parquet, floor with alarmed classmates shuffling out of its reach. The teacher never noticed the commotion and I was too embarrassed to say anything. As a result, I spent an eternally long day in soggy pants and shorts (what a joy that must have been for Mum when I finally got home). Never could I have imagined that, four decades on, I'd be experiencing similar (and far worse) mishaps on a regular basis. Like most people, I had no idea that spinal cord injuries mean far more than not being able to walk.

On that twice-a-day marathon to and from school I'd whinge, drag my feet, scuff my shoes, raise my arms and beg to be carried. Very occasionally, Mum would motivate me with the promise of a treat at the little cake shop halfway home. I'd hover excitedly, outside, obediently holding onto the buggy containing Danny. If she had a few pence to spare, she'd emerge holding out a mini chocolate cake with a flake on the top. It was like birthday and Christmas all at once. If money was tight, it was a gingerbread man. I knew never to moan. I was lucky to get anything.

In 1982, Mum and Dad announced there was a third baby on the way – and we moved to a semi-detached house on Hardy

Mill Road, Harwood. It was only a couple of miles away but a completely different area, with a new school, Harwood Meadows. I can still remember the sheer excitement of Danny and I being shown our new bedroom. It was huge and overlooked a grassy back garden rather than a tiny yard. 'We can play football,' we yelled with delight. In time, I also discovered that nicking from the corner shop and lobbing water balloons were not the done things in Harwood.

Andy arrived that April – making a neat three years between each of us. There were no stories of hunger strikes or withheld toys this time, so I must have accepted this new arrival with good grace. But don't be fooled by the sepia photos of this tight trio, beaming, with our arms draped around each other. We fought like wildcats and we were ultra, and I mean *ultra*-competitive. The Hibbert stubbornness, that determination to come first at all costs, runs through us like a stick of rock. Forget taking part. It's the winning that matters. Even now we're all in our forties and dads ourselves, our Fantasy Football tournaments are brutal. We show no mercy.

When I first met my wife, Gabby, she was shocked at how quickly I ate. And then she met my brothers and it all fell into place. As soon as food appears conversation stops. Bowing over our plates, we tuck in with gusto, keeping senses on high alert for a sneaky fork inching closer. We've all learned to our cost that a split-second blink is long enough for the crispiest roast spud or chip to be swiped from your plate.

We were forever leaping out on each other with a blood-curdling roar. Resulting shrieks, tears or wees of terror from the victim were an added bonus. My favourite prank? Quietly sticking reams of Sellotape across an open doorway then urgently calling my brothers to 'Come quick' so they'd run face first into it (occasionally, an unsuspecting parent would walk into it first which wasn't nearly as hilarious). And we were all football-mad. The new house had a twenty-five-foot living room. With ornaments taken down and furniture pushed back against the walls, it made for a cracking football pitch on rainy afternoons. The bay window at the front of the house was one goal, the patio doors at the back the other. We'd fashion a football out of a load of Sellotape then embark on a riotous game while keeping one wary eye out for the car (we had one by then – much to my delight) pulling onto the drive. There would then ensue an almighty scramble to put everything back in position and take our places, wide-eyed and innocent, over our homework, looking like butter wouldn't melt. Occasionally, we'd be so engrossed in either the game or fighting on the pitch that we wouldn't hear them return and all hell would break loose.

On one occasion, we bravely used a real football. Mum arrived home to a smashed front window, and a trio of tearful boys all blaming each other and begging her not to tell me dad. Somehow, she managed to get it repaired before he came home. But it was tape all the way from then on.

My entire family were ardent Bolton Wanderers supporters. So, I upset the apple cart completely when I rebelled. Dad had taken me to a few games but I hated them. I felt nothing for the ground or the team. United players like Bryan Robson, Gordon Strachan and Jesper Olsen, however, they were like gods. I'd gaze, transfixed, at matches shown on Saturday afternoon telly and beg, cajole, implore Dad to please, please, please take me. I danced for joy when he relented and bought two tickets to an afternoon game against Watford. I remember the clattering of the turnstiles, the smell of chips, the shuffling of boots as we slowly emerged onto the crowded terraces. Above me the Manchester sky was huge. Packed in like sardines, it was noisy, boisterous and bloody brilliant. It felt like coming home. I belonged here. United won 2–0 and it was the best day of my life. I think Dad had hoped that taking me to a crowded game would get it out of my system. But that visit lit the touchpaper and ignited a flame of passion that still burns within me. That Christmas, Santa delivered my first Manchester United kit. It was a bright-blue away strip. I wore it proudly – ignoring the jeers of my Boltonian cousins and uncles. And my bedroom was like a shrine to the team – duvet cover, pillowcase, wallpaper, curtains, lampshade, bin were all red-and-white. I ate, slept and breathed United. Within a few years, I'd earned enough for my own season ticket which I still have to this day.

That pre-match excitement still consumes me. The night before a game, I still lay out my United top, hat and socks. And every single time I enter Old Trafford, either standing tall or in a wheelchair, I turn into that excited seven-year-old with butterflies in my stomach. Not only is my team everything I live and breathe for, I owe the club so much. I've travelled the world to see them play. And I've made the most fantastic friendships – including Mike Burns, who would become like a father to me. And in those dark days after the bombing, I was touched when both players and managers sent recorded video messages urging me to hang in there. I'd ask Gabby to play them over and over.

Both parents were still working long hours and as the eldest I was the man of the house. The familiar 'Look after your brothers' instructions were the bane of my life – particularly if I'd made plans to meet up with me mates for a game of footie. 'Bring your brothers with you,' was the oh-so-simple solution. I'd turn to them and narrow my eyes. Little buggers.

As a result of footie, fisticuffs or horseplay, one of us was always in Bolton Royal Infirmary having stitches or X-rays for broken fingers or toes. I remember Mum saying: 'Bloody hell, they'll be getting social services onto us.' No doubt, we had her pulling her hair out. But teary friends told us at her funeral, 'She never stopped talking about you all and she was so proud of the men you'd become.' It was lovely to hear.

Like every child in Bolton, I learned to ride a bike at Moss Bank Park. Many a stabiliser has been removed on the straight, flat road that cuts right through the park. With grazed hands and bleeding knees, I can still remember the magic of finally keeping my balance on two wheels and zipping along with the wind in my hair (no one wore helmets). After passing my cycling proficiency test at school, my Raleigh Budgie bike (one step below a Chopper, which I yearned for but never got) opened up a whole new world of freedom. I'd make up jam butties, pop them in a rucksack with a packet of crisps (or 'crips', as we called them) and a bottle of Panda Pops then pedal off in search of friends, treasure and adventure. It didn't take much. Finding an old tyre hanging from a tree or rickety old bridge over a stream was like hitting the jackpot and meant hours of play. The only rule was to be back by 7 p.m. for tea. I didn't have a worry or care in the world.

My childhood was a whirlwind of hot summers, freedom and belly laughs, with a few scraps thrown in. When kids from rival estates ventured onto your patch, you learned to stand up for yourself. I was tall for my age and pretty fearless. After one or two initial fights, resulting in the odd bloody nose or thick lip, I was left alone. Not only could I look after myself, I was also a loyal friend and brother – the first to wade in with flailing fists if I got wind that one of them was being picked on.

My maternal grandparents lived about two miles away on a busy little council estate on the edge of Tonge Moor. Grandad Robert 'Bob' Rodie was married to Nanny Jean, who died when I was eleven. It was the first time I'd seem Mum cry and it broke my heart. Bob remarried a few years later and his second wife, Grace, was equally lovely. But I remember enjoying a sense of one-upmanship over my brothers in having known both nannas for longer.

I'd upgraded my bike to a BMX and would fly down to see them along the hairpin corners of the busy Stitch mi Lane. Lord knows how I made it in one piece. Outside 7 Fountains Avenue, grown-ups would sit in faded, stripey deckchairs, putting the world to rights, while kids got up to mischief on the rabbit warren of narrow streets. Inside was even more magical. Entire kitchen drawers were devoted to 'chocolate treats' and there was always a fresh Victoria sponge in the cake tin. There were plug-in electric blankets for sleepovers and crumpled pound notes were pressed into your hand even when it wasn't your birthday or Christmas. Grandad Bob was also the first person we knew to have a SodaStream. An endless supply of American cream soda at the push of a button was the height of luxury and indulgence.

Grandad Bob also introduced me to Ritz crackers and Lancashire cheese. I'd copy the way he ate, catching crumbs in my hand and wiping the corners of my mouth, feeling like such a grown-up. But it wasn't just the treats that lured me there. I hero-worshipped Grandad Bob. Writing this book has made me realise the huge influence he had on me growing up. My beliefs, my principles, how I treat people and want to be treated, in return, is all down to my grandad. The more I talk about him, the prouder and more tearful I become. My mum had a habit of wistfully saying, 'I'm waiting for me ship to come in,' which drove Grandad mad. 'You could be waiting a long time, Janice,' he'd say, in his strong Northern Irish accent, shaking his head. 'It might never come in.' Then he'd turn to me and urge, 'Nothing is ever going to fall into your lap, Martin, lad. Don't wait for your ship to come in. Row out and meet it.' That advice has stood me in good stead – not just financially but emotionally too. 'There will always be bumps in the road, Martin,' Grandad would add. 'You can either sit and mope or you can do something about it.' Those words spurred me on when it came to mastering basic skills like sitting up without vomiting after weeks of lying flat on my back. Without his legacy, I wouldn't be anywhere near the person I am today. He's the backbone that runs through me.

Bob was a pure gentleman. If he caught us Hibbert boys fighting, he'd pull us apart then ensure we 'made up'. 'Even boxers shake hands and hug after a fight,' he'd say wisely. 'Come on, boys. Shake on it.' We always did.

He was exceptionally well-groomed. A beautiful man – he prided himself on his impeccably filed nails and perfectly trimmed moustache. I've always modelled myself on him. On Sunday night, talcumed and in fresh pyjamas after a bath and hair wash, my brothers and I would take it in turns to sit between Mum's knees to have our hair dried. Then we'd get polish and brushes and shine our shoes until you could see your reflection in the toes.

More than anything, Grandad Bob taught me to count my blessings and find happiness in the smallest things. I have a memory of him and Grace happily washing up together, side by side (one washed, one wiped) at their old-fashioned sink, gently swaying to an old Frank Sinatra song. I remember watching wistfully and thinking, I want that. That contentment. That happiness. I still think about my Grandad every single day and miss him so very much. Losing him in 2003 was so very hard and I don't think I've ever truly come to terms with it.

Dad's parents, Bill and Freda, who lived in Hall i' th' Wood, introduced me to my other great love – Laurel and Hardy. Bill and I would sit together on the couch, watching their black-and-white movies, chortling with laughter and re-enacting the mannerisms. I learned to defuse the dodgiest of playground situations with a daft expression or bit of banter. But there were times I took it too far: one afternoon, Grandad Bill was, solemnly, telling us all about his service in the Second World War. 'And, suddenly, we were intercepted by a Fokker plane...'

I couldn't help myself. 'A "fucker"? What's a "fucker plane"?' I chortled, delighting my brothers and earning us all a smart clip around the ear.

Parents evenings and school reports all followed the same lines. 'Martin never, ever, stops talking,' was the exasperated comment from every single teacher. 'Not only is he letting himself down but he's distracting his classmates too.' I couldn't help myself. Both in the classroom and assembly, I'd find myself bursting with the overwhelming urge to comment on anything the teacher said. The only time I wasn't talking was when I was transfixed by the school window-cleaner. I could spend hours contentedly watching a window being soaped and squeegeed. Even now, I love immersing myself in ASMR videos of carpets being cleaned and cars valeted.

It was Grandad Bill who made sense of an occasional, spooky, incident I'd experience as a young child. When we lived in our first house, that little terrace in Tonge Moor, I'd be visited at night by a mystery lady. She'd appear from nowhere at the end of my bed. I'd turn my face to the wall but she'd follow me, gazing inquisitively into my eyes. The hairs on the back of my neck are standing up now just thinking about this. Eventually, I'd hide under the blankets. Next time, I peeped out, she'd be gone. I never shouted for me mum so can't have been scared – just bewildered. The next bit of this story is famous in the Hibbert family. I'm told that I was at Grandad Bill's house, one afternoon, when he got the family photo albums out. 'And here's yer mam and dad on their wedding day,' he said. Apparently, I paid no attention to the bride and groom. Instead, I was fixated on an older woman in the family line-up. I reached out a chubby finger. 'There's that woman!' I said.

My grandad frowned. 'Eh? What you on about?' he asked.

I looked up at him. 'She comes to see me at night,' I'd said, matter-of-factly.

It wasn't often my grandad was lost for words. When he eventually spoke, his voice was shaky. 'That's your guardian angel, lad,' he said. 'She'll always look out for you.' My secret nocturnal visitor was his mum – my great-grandmother, who died years before I was born. I'm convinced that she was there, more than forty years on, watching over me and her great-great-granddaughter, in the Manchester Arena's City Room, when suicide bomber Salman Abedi detonated his device. As we lay dying on the hard, cold, floor I like to picture her looking down on us, shaking her head firmly, and telling me: 'Not yet, Martin. Not yet.'

2

A Grafter

'Martin Hibbert! Get down here NOW!'

The last word ended in a pitch high enough to shatter windows. Steam was erupting from Mum's ears as she stood, hands on hips, at the bottom of the stairs.

'What?' I asked, adopting my best wide-eyed expression. Danny and Andy were hovering behind her. Neither would make eye contact with me.

'Have you been stealing stickers from the corner shop?' she asked through gritted teeth.

I lunged for my brothers. 'You little—'

'… DON'T you blame them,' she continued. 'I have never been so embarrassed in my LIFE.'

Mum had taken them to the Top Shop on the hill in Harwood for a treat after school. Andy had requested 'some of those little stickers that Martin has'. However, the shopkeeper was mystified. 'We don't sell stickers,' he insisted.

'You do! Martin has loads of 'em,' Danny said. 'He said they're 5p each. They're foil aliens and they go a different colour when you hold them up to the light.'

'Ah, you mean the stickers inside the packs of sweet cigarettes. We don't sell them on their own, I'm afraid. You need to buy the sweets.'

Silence hung in the air as the penny dropped; the shopkeeper realised why irate customers had been complaining about sticker-less packs just as Mum finally uncovered my Artful Dodger ways.

'Silly me,' she must have trilled, ushering my protesting brothers out. 'I've just remembered he buys them from a different shop. Bye now!'

I got one hell of a rollicking. The fact that I hadn't taken the sweet ciggies (Yes, they really did sell these back in the '70s!) as well as the stickers didn't count for anything, surprisingly. Nor did my complaint that it wasn't fair that all our school friends were well off – with endless supplies of sweets, superhero comics and shiny stickers that turned a different colour under the light.

Stewing in my room later, feeling particularly hard done by, Grandad Bob's pearls of wisdom rang in my ears. I could sit and moan till the cows came home about the lack of money for treats. Or I could do something about it. I racked my brains for a solution. With my parents working long shifts, me and my brothers already had to do chores around the house. Most kids hate them. Not me. Putting the radio on while getting stuck into housework was my favourite part of the weekend. I'd polish with a yellow duster and a can of Mr Sheen; Danny would hoover and Andy would tidy up. I was brought up on The Beatles, Carpenters and Motown and would belt out the hits with gusto while I worked. Occasionally, Mum would even let me play some of her best vinyl records on the record player. *Saturday Night Fever*, featuring The Bee Gees was a favourite. Within minutes, I'd have abandoned my duties to strut up and down the living room, swinging a tin of paint rifled from the garage, like John Travolta's Tony Manero. Suddenly, I had a brainwave. Rooting under the sink for a bucket and sponge, I pulled my shoulders back, held my head up high and knocked on my neighbour's door.

'Would you like me to wash your car?' I asked.

An hour later, I had soaking wet trainers and two one-pound notes in my fist. By mid-afternoon, I'd earned a tenner. Carefully,

I slotted all but one of the notes into my piggy bank then ran, excitedly, to the Top Shop to buy toffees and a wrestling magazine. I imagine the shopkeeper watched me like a hawk. Knowing I'd earned my treats, as I chewed and turned the pages, made them all the sweeter. 'Well done, Martin,' Mum said proudly. And that was the start of my grafting streak. From then on, I spent every spare minute working. I'd scoff at my brothers; Why sit watching Saturday morning cartoons when you could be making money to buy goodies?

Before each 'shift', I'd stand in front of the hall mirror practising comebacks to rejections. No car? No problem. 'Can I help in the garden, instead, sir? I could sweep up leaves/mow the lawn/tidy your garage?'

Grandad Bob loved hearing about my enterprises. He was a businessman, specialising in turning around failing firms. I hung on his every word about maximising profits and seizing new opportunities. Car washing was just the start. When a local vicar came into our school, recruiting for the church choir, I was jolted out of my customary reverie. *Singers would be paid?* My hand shot up. I had no qualms at all about getting up and performing. I was a cocky little so-and-so with a good set of pipes and was often picked to be the handsome hero in school plays. And the highlight of a rare family holiday in Spain was me singing 'We Are The World' with The Supremes – minus Diana Ross – at our hotel.

The audition, in front of the vicar and choir committee, was like *Britain's Got Talent* (without the raucous audience or sob story). Eyes glistened as my cherubic voice sang. I was in.

I absolutely loved being a choirboy – and not just because I pocketed three pounds for every performance. Two weddings and christenings over a weekend meant twelve pounds. I enjoyed the whole rigmarole of getting dressed up in ruffs and cassocks, practising to perfection, then singing my heart out. It's good for the soul so maybe it was a bit of early therapy. I just know that, for an hour, my voice and spirits soared. And I still know a lot of hymns off by heart, joining in with gusto at weddings and funerals. Perhaps it was also the sense of being part of a community. I've never been good on my own and hate the sound of silence. I need company, the comfort of a background TV show or radio programme.

At eleven, I was old enough to get a paper round at Mo's, the local newsagent. I set my own Big Ben alarm (the old-fashioned kind with a clanging bell that would wake the dead) at 6.30 a.m. weekdays and at 7 a.m. on a Saturday. I'd swell with pride hearing Mo tell customers I was the best paperboy he'd ever had. And the oldest. I only stopped when I went to university! I took my responsibilities very seriously. In seven years, I never had a single day off sick, delivering my papers in hail, rain or blazing sunshine. My customers, who I always called 'sir' and 'madam', relied on me. I couldn't let them down. I'd fold the papers carefully so that they'd open out beautifully with minimal creases.

One old dear would leave her door open so I could shelter from the rain and have a cup of tea with her. As Christmas approached, I couldn't stand the thought of tips being shared out amongst all the paperboys who weren't half as conscientious or reliable as I was. I wrote personalised cards to each customer – wishing them a lovely Christmas from their paperboy, Martin, and telling them how much I enjoyed delivering their paper each day. Next day, there'd be a fiver or a tenner waiting for me: I wasn't just a paperboy – I was a businessman, just like Grandad Bob. A freemason, he was always immaculately dressed in a suit, tie and cap.

With my first wages, I bought myself a smart shirt and tie so I could look just like Bob. I wore my new grown-up clobber to meet up with my friends in town. Clad in their jeans and T-shirts, they looked me up and down in astonishment. 'What the hell are you wearing, Hibbert, you dickhead?' they scoffed.

'Laugh as much as you want,' I shrugged. My grandad was cool and I was cool. End of. I cringe at the memory but part of me admires young Martin. And to this day, if I like something, I'll wear it – regardless of whether it's high fashion or not.

Mum's regular trips to the cash-and-carry triggered yet another money-making scheme. One week she let me and my best friend Richard Northrop tag along. Pooling our paper-round money we chose giant sweetshop jars of midget gems, cola cubes and cough candy twists and paper bags. Back in the kitchen, we used Mum's weighing scales to carefully measure out quarter-pound bags of sweets to sell at school. Each day, we'd do a recce of tuck shop prices – then undercut them. 'We'll be selling in the science lab at breaktime – pass it on,' we'd whisper during lessons. I sold the merchandise, while Richard kept a careful lookout for patrolling teachers. I'd be totting up, professionally, while kids thronged around us clutching hot fistfuls of coins.

Running for the bus at home time, we'd literally jingle from all the loose change in our bags and pockets. With our profits we expanded into crisps and chocolate bars – and even bought a Helix lockable cash box for takings! It was a proper little empire.

One morning, I went into Mo's bright and early for my papers, and stopped dead in front of his latest display. 'What is *this*?' I breathed, transfixed.

He beamed at my reaction. 'It's the latest thing, Martin,' he said.

There was a pause. 'I'll take 'em all,' I said decisively.

I cleared out Mo's entire stock of mini cans of pop that he'd only just unpacked from the warehouse. Our rucksacks weighed a ton going into school that morning but I remember rubbing my hands in anticipation. 'These'll fly off,' I said to Richard. And I was right. We couldn't get them out of our bags quick enough. After buying them for 15p each, we sold them for 50p.

Ski-patterned jumpers were the height of fashion that winter. After school, I caught a bus straight into town and bought two in different colours – emptying my bulging pockets of change onto the counter. By now, my profits easily covered tickets to see my beloved Manchester United. Wearing my favourite hat and scarf and the latest kit, I'd strut confidently through Salford to and from games. Grown men would hesitate to venture, alone, in that area these days but I honestly don't remember ever being scared of anyone or anything.

At fifteen, I also got an evening job washing up at Egerton House Hotel in Blackburn Road. (I've no idea how I worked all those hours and still did well at school.) I'd carefully watch the chefs as they worked and, before long, they'd roped me in to help them. I loved wearing chef whites and learning to effortlessly slice mushrooms and peppers with heavy, professional knives and cook steaks on a sizzling griddle. Even better was tucking into food together once the restaurant was closed.

Before long, I'd bought a season ticket at Old Trafford. It felt like gold in my hand. My own seat! I really had made it. Years of working and learning from Grandad Bob had given me a confidence beyond my years. I turned to the gentleman beside me. 'Hello, sir, I'm Martin. Nice to meet you,' I said, reaching out my hand.

'Hello, young man. I'm Mike,' he replied, shaking my hand firmly. We beamed at each other. 'And this,' said Mike Burns, gesturing to the man beside him, 'is Jon the shoe' (Jon was a cobbler – hence his name. Men were often known for their trade). From that moment on we were inseparable at games. Mike, in particularly, became a father figure as we travelled all over Europe to watch the team in tournaments. We'd take in the game then spend a few days sightseeing.

Mike lived in Lichfield with his wife, Jackie, and would invite me down to visit. The first time I went for dinner, Jackie served fajitas – plonking a big bowl of spiced chicken in front of me. Used to eating quickly, I tucked in ravenously wondering, occasionally, why no one else had started. It was only when I'd finished the last crammed wrap I realised neither of them had eaten a thing – and there was no other bowl on the table. I'd polished off the lot! Another time, I scoffed my way through an entire bowl of fruit while I stood in the kitchen yakking. It was a standing joke that I'd demolish any food within reaching distance. Each evening, we'd sit and chat – putting the world to rights. And next morning, Mike would treat me to his famous Burnsey Breakfast – a big fry-up with all the trimmings. I've been blessed to have met some amazing people in my life who bring out the best. And Mike was one of them.

After doing well in my GCSEs I enrolled in a BTEC in business studies and finance at Bolton College. With the memory of those long, wet, miserable walks to our first school still fresh in my mind, I was counting down the days to my seventeenth birthday so that I could make the journey by car. I was far too impatient for weekly driving lessons. That would take for ever. Instead, I went halves on a week-long, intense course during the summer holidays, passing my test on the final day. The first thing I did was fulfil a long-standing promise to Grandad Bob. Even as a small child I'd tell him, 'Just you wait, Grandad. You won't have to get the bus home from bowling. I'll drive you in my car.'

OK, it was my mum's white Ford Escort, forever conking out, that I turned up in that day. But Grandad was just as proud. 'This is my grandson, Martin,' he told his teammates, as I pulled up. 'He's driving now, you know!'

I loved getting behind the wheel – and still do. Mum put me on her insurance and I'd get up at stupid o'clock to drive her to work so that I could have her car for the rest of the day. I'd pick my mates up – for a charge, of course. When Mum upgraded to a red Nova, I jazzed it up with sporty accessories to make it look a bit more like a sports car. She didn't even notice!

Throughout college, I continued my morning paper round and washing up in the evenings. While my friends were out drinking and partying, I was working every night – bringing home six hundred pounds a month.

At eighteen, I got a distinction in my BTEC and moved to Hull University to do business studies. I did well in my course and, early on, found yet another way to eke out my student grant, having given up my paper round and restaurant job.

Working in the restaurant had turned me into a confident cook. I'd stock up in Kwik Save then spend hours rustling up stir fries, curries and casseroles which I'd flog to fellow students. Then I'd leave them to it and head to the pub for best steak and chips with my takings!

Just before the end of the first year, disaster struck. Things hadn't been great between Mum and Dad for years. Now they were separating and it was far from amicable. I pulled my battered suitcase out from under the bed. Mum and the boys needed me. I was going home. I'd never really fitted in with university life. I missed me mum, me friends, the Manchester United games. I'd joined a supporters' club and would still attend matches with Mike and The Shoe but I felt a pang every time the coach pulled away from Old Trafford. I'd even missed me brothers! Mum protested weakly but, I think, secretly she was relieved I was back. Andy reminded me recently that, on that first night back home, I'd stood up after tea and made a dramatic speech. 'We're Hibberts and we'll survive,' I announced, pulling everyone in for a rare group hug. Mum had turned to me, eyes glistening. 'You're the man of the house now, Martin,' she said.

With the boys still at school and bills piling up it was clear Mum was struggling. It broke our hearts to sell the family home but we had no choice, downsizing to a smaller house on Hazelwood Avenue, still in Harwood. I applied for three jobs in banking – and got them all – accepting a teller position with Barclays in the St Ann's Square city centre branch. I hit it off from day one. Chatting to customers and being part of a team was the perfect job for me. I loved the buzz when famous actors and footballers came to the branch. My talking skills hadn't diminished with age. Occasionally, I'd hear a cough from my manager and realise a queue was snaking out of the door. Back home, I'd contribute to bills, cook dinner for the family and make the boys' packed lunches for the following day. Danny's reminded me that I even bought him a kitten to lift his spirits.

After a couple of years on the counter, you could progress down either the retail or business route. I'd set my heart on looking after the footballers' accounts only to be told, 'We're not sure private banking's for you because of your strong accent'. There were no discrimination laws back then. But rather than being affronted, I saw it as a challenge and worked all the harder to prove myself. By 2000, I was an account executive looking after accounts for footballers and the rich and famous. This was where I'd wanted to be. It was like the SAS of banking. I felt like a king.

Aged nineteen, a bit late to the dating scene, I started going out with Sarah, a fellow cashier. Relationships were frowned upon so she moved to another branch so we could keep seeing each other. We marked the millennium by buying our first house. The following year we discovered we were going to be parents. It was a bit sooner than we'd planned (I was only twenty-five) but we were over the moon. I was more nervous breaking the news to Mike than I was telling my own parents. He was quite a religious person and I think he was a bit upset that we were having a child before getting married. But he congratulated me and we sat up having our usual brandy once everyone else had gone to bed. His opinion really mattered to me. It was only afterwards he confessed he was worried sick at how I'd manage fatherhood!

Thankfully, Sarah had a textbook pregnancy. I took time off work to attend every single antenatal appointment and birth preparation class with her. We were keen to find out if we were having a boy or girl but, at the twenty-week scan our baby positioned itself in such a way that the sonographer couldn't tell us. We decided on a water birth at Bolton Royal Infirmary and I can still remember the awe and wonder I felt as Sarah pushed our baby into the world on 9 October 2002. She weighed 7 lb on the dot – just as I'd done.

'It's a girl,' someone cried. In the final moments of childbirth Sarah suffered complications and needed to be whisked away for surgery. I was shell-shocked as the umbilical cord was quickly clamped before this wriggling, furious, bundle of life – fresh and warm from the womb – was placed directly into my arms. As advised by the midwife, I'd taken my T-shirt off first for that early, precious skin-to-skin contact. It was astonishing. For so long I'd been talking to this growing bump – marvelling at the indentations of a heel or elbow as it kicked and squirmed in response inside Sarah's tummy. And now, there was a real-life baby in my arms. I've never shared this detail but, deep down, I'd been hoping for a boy – and imagining footy in the park, kickabouts and sharing the joy of Man United.

But suddenly it happened. My baby girl stopped crying and gazed up at me with these solemn, dark, unblinking eyes. As her tiny perfect fingers folded over my index finger. I felt a stirring within me like nothing I'd ever felt before. It was love. Pure, undiluted love. *My girl. My beautiful girl.*

We'd already chosen names. There'd been a girl at primary school called Eve Mercer (now Simms) – and I'd always loved the name. Our baby's second name? Victoria, of course, after David Beckham's wife.

'Hello Eve,' I whispered, choking back tears. 'It's me… Daddy.' Then I stroked her still-damp, blonde, downy hair and lowered my head to plant a kiss on her velvety soft forehead. I knew in that moment I would do anything… *anything*, to look after her, protect her and keep her safe.

3

Highs and Increasing Lows

The twenty-second of May 2017 should have been the date inscribed on my gravestone. That was the night that I lay dying on the hard, cold floor of Manchester Arena's City Room, a few feet away from my daughter. She, too, was barely clinging to life. We were the closest survivors to the bomber to survive. As you can imagine, our injuries were horrific. Life-changing in so many ways.

As you'll read further in this book it's a miracle that either – let alone both – of us survived. But one thing I haven't spoken widely about is how the night of the bombing wasn't the first time my life came close to ending. I'd come terrifyingly close just four months earlier. And on that occasion, it wasn't down to the crazed actions of a deranged terrorist. It was entirely down to me. Looking back now, it's hard to imagine that that cocky young man, who had everything to live for – a wife and child, family and friends who loved him, would even contemplate suicide, let alone plan it right down to the last detail. But that's depression for you. It's a period in my life that's painful to recall but I feel I need to share it. It may go some way to explaining how I coped with the horror that Salman Abedi unleashed just four months later at the Ariana Grande concert. And if it encourages others, feeling total and utter despair, to reach out for help, then it will be worth it. So here goes…

Back in September 2002, I had no idea what lay ahead. Like all new parents, we were shocked to discover there was no manual for looking after a baby. After the initial excitement of leaving hospital as a family, I remember the overwhelming sense of blind panic that engulfed us as we closed the front door, looked at Eve sleeping peacefully in her car seat and realised that we were responsible for keeping this little human alive. It didn't help that, when Eve woke, she started crying... and never stopped. Days and nights blurred into one. We became stupefied, then zombified, with lack of sleep. Lord knows how I functioned at work. Eventually, our mums hatched an intervention plan and whisked Eve away, with supplies of expressed milk, so that we could get some much needed sleep. But they were back all too soon – with a still-screaming baby. In desperation, we sought medical help and discovered Eve was lactose intolerant. As soon as we switched her to special formula (it definitely was special – twenty quid a pot!), things calmed down. She was perfect.

I knew the type of dad I wanted to be and, with good people like Mike and Grandad Bob around me I was able to be that person. With both Sarah and I working, Eve was looked after by Sarah's mum. We delightedly ticked off milestones: first tooth, first solid food, first word, first tentative, wobbly steps on tiny feet...

Both sets of great grandparents absolutely doted on her. It was lovely to see their faces light up when we visited. On her first birthday, I brought my little girl into work to meet everyone. She buried her face into my chest, occasionally looking around to smile shyly. I couldn't have been prouder – or happier. People say you turn into a man at eighteen but I don't agree. You turn into a man when you become a dad.

'I was worried when you said you were having a baby,' Mike confessed afterwards. 'You were cocky and arrogant and I genuinely didn't think you were ready.' *Er, cheers mate!* He'd had terrible visions of me trying to feed a newborn baby pizza, kebabs and Mars Bars. 'I'm not often proven wrong, Martin,' he said. 'But the change in you has been incredible and you're an amazing dad. I'm proud of you.' I was so choked, I couldn't speak.

Over time, people inevitably asked when we'd be giving her a sibling. But the thought never crossed our minds. Eve genuinely felt enough. But, also, we couldn't afford to have another child, especially when Sarah's parents, who had been looking after Eve while we worked, moved away when her dad was promoted. Overnight, we had huge nursery bills to pay on top of our existing outgoings. I'd been chipping in to help Mum and had nothing in the way of savings. We were struggling to keep our heads above water.

Bank employees weren't allowed overdrafts or to have financial issues. As a temporary measure we started using credit cards – only to panic when the bills came in. My brothers and parents would occasionally bail us out – only for us to realise we couldn't pay them back. Looking back, I'm mortified at how the situation escalated and how I let people down. I owe everything to an understanding boss, Scott Wheble, who sat me down, went through my finances and put us in touch with people who helped us get back on an even keel.

In the current cost of living crisis, my heart goes out to people struggling. Yes, there's more to life than money. But when you don't have it, it matters a great deal, seeping into every aspect of your life, turning the tiniest hairline crack in a relationship into a great, wide, chasm. When Eve was fifteen months old, things unravelled further on the night of our work Christmas party. It was a black-tie do and, after months of patiently growing my hair, it was long enough to wear in David Beckham's samurai warrior style – long, with a section tied up on top. Trust me, it was a good look at the time. I felt a million dollars. Andy dropped us off in my car and agreed to pick us up later, for a fee – he'd learned from the best! Halfway through the dinner, I noticed a missed call from Mum, who was babysitting.

'It's fine, love,' she insisted when I rang her back. 'Enjoy your evening.'

On the way home, Andy was unusually quiet. Mum answered the front door, red-eyed. Her face crumpled. 'I'm sorry, love,' she wept. 'I didn't want to spoil your evening. But your grandad died this evening.'

As a wave of grief washed over me my knees buckled and I sank to the ground. Kneeling in despair, I buried my face in my hands and cried. *Grandad. Grandad.* He hadn't been feeling well earlier that evening and had been admitted to Bolton Royal Infirmary but died a few hours later. Suddenly, I'd scrambled to my feet. 'I need to see him,' I said. My best shoes clicked as we made our way towards the hospital mortuary. Even then I was convinced he wouldn't be there. It was all a big mistake. Grandad couldn't be dead! It was surreal seeing him lying there looking for all the world like he was sleeping. Stooping down, I kissed his cold, waxy forehead. Hot tears spilled onto his face as I thanked him for being in my life and told him how much I loved him and would miss him. Then I whispered words that I have never shared with anyone. I'm not religious but, in the stillness of that room, I had the overwhelming sense that he was still there. That he could hear me. The thought of never hearing from him again was unbearable. But, if he wanted to reach out to me from the other side, and I heard those exact words repeated back to me, I'd know it really was Grandad.

The coffin weighed a ton as we hoisted it onto our shoulders. 'Bloody hell, has he got his bowling balls in there with him?' I remember hissing to Danny and Andy. Standing up to give a reading almost finished me off but, choking back tears, I did it. Afterwards Nanna Grace hugged me. 'Your Grandad was always so proud of you, Martin,' she said. I let the tears flow as I hugged her. A little bit of sunshine had gone from my life. And I'd never get it back.

Grandad Bob had enjoyed a year with Eve, which I'm grateful for. But my life seemed so empty without him. We were stunned when doctors listed the cause of death as asbestosis – a serious lung condition triggered by exposure to asbestos. We had no idea he was even ill.

Sarah and I drifted apart. The years passed until, heartbroken, we agreed to call it a day. Because we weren't married, the legal situation was complicated and took for ever to sort. But we worked out an arrangement whereby I'd move back in with Mum and have Eve at weekends. In July 2009, shortly before Eve's seventh birthday, I packed my bags, left my key on the hallway table and closed the front door behind me for good. I cried all the way to Mum's. Not having Eve in my life every day broke me. It was like a bereavement. I lived for Fridays, for the moment I hovered, excitedly, at the school gate waiting for the bell so I could scoop her up in my arms. 'Daddy!' she'd shriek, hurtling towards me.

The next two days would be a whirlwind of birthday parties, playdates, trips to the cinema, film nights snuggled on the sofa with popcorn or hours at the playground. As Eve grew older, she shared my love of music and I took her to her first ever concert to see JLS. I hoped that Eve would also share my love for United and was gutted when she confessed that she'd hated her first game. It was noisy, too crowded and boring, apparently. 'You go Daddy – and I'll stay with Nana.' I'd hurry home before the final whistle to spend more time with her.

From Sunday lunchtime, as the countdown started for her return to Sarah, my mood would start to drop. Driving her back, kissing her goodbye for another five days, was soul-destroying. Sometimes, I was so upset Mum would do the return for me. Monday mornings with another Eve-less week stretching out ahead of me were unbearable.

I had no interest in meeting another partner. All I wanted was to get my head down, do my job well, and enjoy Eve at the weekends. Thank heavens, I had brilliant friends who kept me going. Karl Pemberton was one of the first friends I made at RBS in 2007 and I met Steve Lloyd through private banking two years later. He's fifteen years older than me but when you share a love of Marvel films any age gap melts away.

Two years before splitting with Sarah, I'd been promoted to a new job with RBS in Bradford. It meant an hour's commute each day from Bolton to Bradford. As I was to learn, an hour is a long time with dark thoughts whirling around your mind. Over time, I found myself looking out for a colleague who worked on the floor above. I only caught occasional glimpses of Gabby but she was petite, blonde, and stunning. One Friday some workmates arranged a lunchtime drink and fixed it for her to be there as well. It was sod's law that an important call from a client came through just as I was due to leave. I was still on the phone when they all traipsed back. I felt wretched all afternoon. What on earth would she think?

At home time, I spotted her heading for the car park. Sprinting out, I tapped on her window just as she was reversing out of her space – nearly giving her a heart attack. We joke now that I leaped on her bonnet like Bodie and Doyle rolling across cars in *The Professionals*. 'I'm really sorry about today,' I blurted. 'I really want to take you out. Here's my card. Drop me a message and we'll do lunch or something.' How cocky is that? Putting the onus on her to call me.

With a smile, she took the card, then flushed as she noticed me glancing into the back of her car. 'Ignore the logs – I'm off to the tip at the weekend,' she said, before closing the window. Logs? They were trees! Trees and twigs – filling every spare inch of the interior. I swear blind now that she'd been driving around with them for six months. Knowing Gabby as I do now it wouldn't have surprised me in the slightest.

She bided her time before messaging me. And a week later, we had our first date at the Shibden Mill Inn. There were no awkward silences while cutlery scraped plates. It was as if we'd known each other for ever. Driving home from our second date, at a restaurant in Harrogate, I decided to play my favourite song for her. 'It's quite unusual,' I warned. As the haunting melody began her smile froze. She turned to look at me in astonishment, then quickly turned away. 'Gabby?' I ventured.

Silence. Leaning forward, I was horrified to see her biting her lip, trying in vain to stop tears spilling down her face. Oh God, what? I thought, reaching for the dial. Was it played at a parent's funeral? Did it trigger traumatic memories? But she reached out to stop me and gave a watery smile. 'I haven't heard this version before. But this is my favourite song,' she said.

It was an a cappella version of Kate Bush's 'This Woman's Work' by an artist called Maxwell. It's utterly beautiful. Mum used to say, 'If you just hear the tune, you're doing it wrong. You need to immerse yourself in it – really feel the meaning behind the melody and the lyrics.' The music washed over us and, wordlessly, our outstretched hands met. In that moment, we knew we'd found each other.

Nervously, I took Gabby to meet Mike and he gave her the seal of approval. In 2010, I moved into her Bradford home. Each Friday I'd still pick up Eve from school and spend the weekend with her at Mum's in Bolton. I longed for Gabby to share my love for United and took her to the semi-final of the Champions League against Chelsea. She was the only woman in a sea of men. There was a massive surge from behind when they came close to scoring and her glasses nearly flew off in the melee. 'It's not for me, love,' she confessed afterwards. I was gutted that the two women in my life didn't share this incredible passion.

In 2012, we discovered Gabby, then thirty-nine, was pregnant. We told our mums and best friends but otherwise kept it secret. 'Not until the three-month scan,' we decided. I couldn't wait to tell Eve she was going to be a big sister.

'This might feel a little cold,' the sonographer said, squirting gel onto Gabby's exposed tummy. We were at Bradford Royal Infirmary for the twelve-week scan. I held her hand as we gazed at the monitor, waiting for a flicker of life to appear. The sonographer stared intently at the screen as she gently slid the probe over Gabby's abdomen. Then she put the probe down. 'I'm just going to fetch a colleague,' she said, leaving the room.

Shit.

Gabby and I looked at each other, then back at the screen. Neither of us uttered a word. With the first scan with Eve, they'd found her straight away. The sonographer returned with a consultant. More gel. More probing. And then the words 'I'm sorry.' The baby had never formed properly. There was no heartbeat. Just an empty sac. Numb and dry-eyed with shock, we were led to another room where an appointment was made for Gabby to have a dilation and curettage procedure to remove the remains of the pregnancy from her uterus. Gabby clutched her appointment card. Neither of us said a word all the way home. What was there to say? I'd never felt so helpless in my life.

Next day, I was due to take Eve out. 'You go, I'll be fine, honestly,' Gabby said.

I'd had it all worked out: handing Eve an envelope and grinning as she pulled out the scan photo. Now, my biggest job was to hide my sadness. Later that afternoon, my mobile rang. It was Gabby – in so much pain from contractions she could barely speak. 'I don't know what to do,' she whimpered. 'I've tried the hospital department but there's no answer.' Then she cried out as another came. 'Martin, it's getting worse. I'm frightened.'

I left Eve with Mum and raced home to find Gabby on the floor, unable to move. Paramedics arrived just as I was about to carry her to the car. She needed gulps of oxygen just to get into the ambulance. At Bradford Royal Infirmary, Gabby was given painkillers and admitted to a private room on the maternity ward. At least, there, with the door shut, she wouldn't be able to hear the cries of newborn babies. I cuddled up behind her on the bed and we lay like that, all night, drifting into fitful sleep. Next morning, pale and scared, she was wheeled to theatre. Very few people knew about the miscarriage. That was the way Gabby wanted it. She was back at work a week later – desperate to take her mind off it.

When we felt stronger, we agreed that if it happened again, fine, but we wouldn't actively try to get pregnant. It was never a huge issue. We had each other. For Easter 2012, I booked a weekend away for us in Barcelona. While watching a United game in a pub I downed four pints for Dutch courage. Afterwards, a bit squiffy, we visited the cathedral. And there, in a prayer room of the cathedral, I got down on one knee and asked this incredible woman to marry me. Caught up in nerves I hadn't realised it was 1 April. Thank heavens, Gabby took me seriously and said, 'Yes.'

Life was good. I had a daughter I adored. A fiancée I loved. A wedding on the horizon. The job I'd hankered after. So why did black moods descend on me? I came to dread the lone motorway drives on Friday and Sunday evening after dropping off Eve. Because that's when the dark thoughts would descend.

You're a rubbish dad. A terrible fiancé. You're bad at your job. No one likes you.

I'd turn the radio up, trying to drown them out. But they just grew louder. I'd arrive at my destination a trembling wreck, soaked with cold, clammy sweat. Then I'd take a deep breath, put my smiling mask on and get ready to give an Oscar-winning performance of happy-go-lucky, easy-come-easy-go Martin. For months I managed to hide it. But Gabby knew something was up. 'Is everything OK? Are *we* OK?' she'd ask, with a worried expression. 'You don't seem your usual self.' But I assured her I was just tired. Busy at work. One Saturday lunchtime, she came into the kitchen. 'You'll be late for the game if you don't get going,' she said.

'I'm not going,' I said blankly. 'Don't feel like it.'

She stared at me in disbelief. 'OK, who are you? And what have you done with the real Martin Hibbert?' she joked. I didn't laugh. Later she found me in bed, curtains drawn, staring blankly at the ceiling. 'Martin,' she ventured, 'what's wrong?'

As I blinked, tears trickled from my eyes and seeped into the pillow. 'I don't know,' I whispered. I assured Gabby I loved her. I wanted to marry her. But I was becoming consumed with this overwhelming feeling of despair and panic. At work, I'd stare at the ringing phone on my desk, unable to physically answer it. I couldn't sleep, I couldn't eat. I'd wake in the early hours panicking over what new catastrophes the day would bring. I'd try to rehearse what I'd say or do. My mind was constantly whirling. It was exhausting. I'd always taken such pride in my appearance. Now, I wore crumpled shirts. Stopped polishing my shoes. Went longer without shaving.

I could see the worry in Gabby's face. But I assured her it was just a blip. One of my clients, Alison, was a GP. When we met to discuss her finances, she'd look at me intently and ask if I was OK. Soon afterwards, I read an article in which a former, well-known, premier footballer revealed his battle with clinical depression. My eyes devoured the words, reading of the lethargy, despair, self-loathing, suicidal thoughts… *Oh my God. That's me.* I rang Alison on the pretence of talking about her account. But as soon as I heard her voice I burst into tears. 'Martin?' she asked gently. 'Are you OK?'

I could barely get the words out. 'I've read an interview with Stan Collymore and I think it's me. I'm like this all the time,' I gabbled. 'I feel like I'm losing my mind. I just don't know who I am. I feel like Clark Kent in *Superman III* when he's two different people. When I look in the mirror it's not me I'm seeing. I feel like I'm inside a bad version of me and I can't get out. I just want to scream all the time. *I'm not me!*'

She listened patiently. 'I think you need to see a GP, Martin,' she said gently. 'Please make an appointment today.'

My head was spinning. 'But how can I have depression? I've nothing to be depressed about. I'm about to get married. I love Gabby. And I love my daughter.'

Alison patiently explained that it wasn't a case of 'pulling myself together' or 'counting blessings'. Clinical depression was a mental illness. And I needed professional help. I booked an appointment for first thing next morning. I can smile now at the doctor's confused face when I used the *Superman III* analogy. 'Erm, I haven't seen that one,' he admitted. But he did diagnose depression and prescribed medication. I cried all the way back to work, dreading telling my line managers. I was terrified of their reaction. Would they fire me on the spot? Say I wasn't up to the job? They didn't. But they weren't brimming over with understanding, either. I don't blame them in the slightest. It's only in the last few years that people have really opened up about mental illness.

'Don't be daft,' one scoffed. 'You're just stressed with the wedding plans.'

Others couldn't hide their bemusement. 'You? Depression? Don't be ridiculous.' I forced a smile. 'Yeah, you're right. Doctors, eh?'

Those next few weeks, waiting for the 'happy pills' to kick in was a horrendous time. But gradually, slowly, the despair softened around the edges. The black cloud turned to grey. The panics eased. The voices quietened. When I looked in the mirror I saw me again. I wasn't cured. But I was a heck of a lot better than I was.

The twenty-third of August 2014 was, after Eve's birth, the happiest day of my life. We were married at the Inn At Whitewell in the Forest of Bowland. One of my favourite photos is of Eve, one of the bridesmaids, wrapping her arms around Gabby's waist and hugging her tightly. *My two girls.* Mike was my best man, standing proudly beside me and solemnly handing over the rings. I'd come a long way from the cocky, know-it-all kid of sixteen he'd first met at Old Trafford. Now, I was thirty-seven. A proper grown-up.

I led Gabby on to the floor for our first dance – the song I'd played on our second date. It's not the easiest song to dance to. It was more of a shuffle, really, as we gazed goofily into each other's eyes. You could see some of our seventy-five guests exchanging *'weird song'* glances. But we didn't care. That song means the world to us.

We had a wonderful honeymoon in St Lucia in the Caribbean, in a beachside apartment with a butler waiting on us hand and foot. It was a magical time. Back home, we settled down to married life. Through that winter, I noticed my moods darkening again. The doctor increased the dose of the medication but it made little difference. 'I'll be all right,' I assured Gabby. 'It's just the dark nights and mornings.'

If anyone had told me how bad things would get, I would never, ever, have believed them.

4

Hitting Rock Bottom

By 2016, four years after the miscarriage, we'd accepted a baby wasn't going to happen. We decided on the next best thing. A puppy. We already had our girl, Eve. A boy dog would make our family complete. We chose the name, Alfie, and set our hearts on a blue roan cocker spaniel – along with, it seemed, everyone else in the north-west. Puppies were being snapped up before they were even born.

I left my details with so many people and was in a meeting when a call came from Manchester. A litter had just become available. 'I'm on my way,' I said, before he'd even finished speaking. Abruptly drawing the meeting to a close, I virtually skipped to my car.

The majority of the pups were bitches, with just two boys. One of them left the melee of play-fighting with his siblings and scampered straight over to me. I gently scooped him up and felt my heart melt as this bundle of warm softness settled into my arms and nuzzled me. He was jet-black, apart from some paler markings down his nose and around his muzzle. Lifting him up under his two front legs, I held him in front of me so that our faces were an inch apart. A little pink tongue licked my nose. Then, as his rich, chocolate-brown eyes gazed into mine, I could swear he could see into my very soul. 'Hello, Alfie,' I said. Nestling him back into the crook of my arm, I pulled my phone out and with one, fumbling, hand rang Gabby. 'I've found him! I've found our dog.'

I turned to the owner. 'I'll have him, please.'

The man grimaced. 'No can do, I'm afraid. They go on sale on Saturday – first come first served.'

I reached for my bank card. 'Can I reserve him? Pay a deposit?' The answer was a firm no. 'I'm really sorry but they're not for sale until then,' he said apologetically.

I kissed the top of Alfie's soft black head then, reluctantly, placed him back in the pen. He looked up at me with a beseeching expression. 'What time do you open Saturday?' I sighed.

We set the alarm extra early at the weekend, terrified of finding a massive queue outside the shop. 'Honestly, he's a beauty – everyone will want him,' I said to Gabby. We got there to find the street deserted. Yes! Finally, there was a jangling of keys and the poor manager was nearly knocked down in our eagerness to reach Alfie. There was a flurry of excited yelps from the puppy pen as we hurried towards it. And there he was, standing on his back legs, resting his front paws up against the edge of the pen. Our boy. I scooped him up tenderly and, like a proud dad, showed him to Gabby. 'He's gorgeous,' she breathed, reaching out to stroke his velvety soft ears. She cuddled him while I paid five hundred pounds.

'Right, he's ready for you,' said the manager, handing over paperwork.

Gabby and I exchanged alarmed looks. 'Erm, don't we pick him up in a few days?' I asked. 'We haven't even got a collar!'

He smiled and started writing out a shopping list. Gabby stayed with Alfie while I dashed to the pet shop and spent the best part of a grand on a crate, dog bed, training pads, blankets, towels, bowls, toys, balls, collar, lead, harness, identity tag...

We'd agreed Alfie would sleep downstairs in his crate. But after just a few minutes of his pitiful whimpers, whines, howls and yelps, Gabby sat up. 'I can't bear it,' she said, throwing back the duvet and hurrying downstairs. She returned with a delighted Alfie in her arms. 'Just for tonight,' she said, nestling him on the bed. He's slept there ever since. Much to her annoyance, Alfie became 'my boy', my shadow. Wherever I was, Alfie was two paces behind. If I was busy on my laptop, he'd sit by my feet, resting his head on his paws but keeping a faithful gaze on me.

At this time, I was nurturing plans to leave banking and set up my own business – as a sporting agent for footballer players. I hoped my new activities would distract me from the disquiet that was bubbling away again inside my head. It started as a sense of unease that something wasn't quite right. Then it became a whisper, a swirl. It was back. And it was stronger this time.

I went back to my GP. 'The tablets have stopped working,' I said. We tried countless medications. But nothing provided relief. The bad/evil Superman analogy is the most accurate description. In the film, Superman temporarily becomes two separate beings after being exposed to synthetic kryptonite. I felt like I was being controlled, taken over, consumed by 'Bad/Sad Martin' – a negative, miserable, hateful version of myself.

With each day that passed Bad (although strictly speaking he wasn't bad, just very unhappy, low and angry)/Sad Martin was taking possession of more cells, more fibres of my being. He delighted in telling Good Martin that he was useless, pathetic, a waste of space, hated by everyone. *You're a crap father,* he'd goad and gloat. *Gabby regrets ever marrying you. Your friends only pretend to like you. They hate you really.* I tried to bat the words off. But it was a relentless deluge. It's all I heard, day and night.

In desperation, I threw myself into business plans and finding things to do with Eve, Gabby and Alfie. I'd plaster a smile on my face. Have the radio and TV playing excessively loud. Did everything I could to silence the voices in my head. But on those frequent motorway drives to see Eve, they'd reach a crescendo. I became obsessed by one particular bridge on the M62. There was a long straight length of motorway leading up to it. *Plenty of time to put your foot down and keep it there, Bad/Sad Martin would suggest.*

The bridge became like a siren, luring me towards it. As I approached it, I'd start sweating as a compulsive urge to sharply yank the steering wheel to the right and plough straight into it, rose up within me. At times, I'd have to put my hazard lights on and – shaking, sweating, crying – pull over onto the hard shoulder until the moment had passed. I was literally fighting the baddie inside me. I'd already broken down in front of both Mum and Gabby and confessed how bad things were. But I assured them that I'd be OK. It was temporary. The tablets would kick in soon. It would pass. Christmas was on the horizon.

On Christmas Day 2016 I had a special present for Eve to open. 'Oooh – an Ariana Grande calendar,' she exclaimed as she tore open the paper. 'Thanks, Daddy.'

I grinned. She didn't suspect a thing. 'Turn to May,' I suggested. 'See what's there.'

Intrigued, she flipped through the months until she found May. Monday the twenty-second leapt out of the page – highlighted, circled and covered in stars. Meanwhile, I'd pulled off my Christmas jumper with a flourish. 'What's on 22 May?' she asked, frowning. 'And what on earth are you wearing?' she laughed at my 'Ariana Grande is my Girlfriend' T-shirt.

'Now, I wonder what it could be…?' I said thoughtfully. 'I wonder if there might be any clues in the back pocket of the calendar…?'

Quick as a flash, Eve flicked to the back cover, rooted inside the document compartment and pulled out two tickets. Her eyes widened as she scanned the details. *Dangerous Woman tour, Manchester Arena, 22 May, VIP private box.*

'OH MY GOD!' she shrieked, jumping up and down. Then she threw her arms around me and planted a flurry of kisses on my cheek. 'You said they were sold out! Thank you. Thank you. Thank you. This is the best present ever.'

Gabby and I exchanged grins over her head. *Well, that went down well.* Eve had been begging for tickets for the concert when they went on sale two months earlier. The show in Manchester was the only one in the north of England and they'd been snapped up by fans from as far afield as Scotland. Then I'd remembered a client who rented a VIP box at the arena. He agreed to sell me two seats for his front row for £150 each.

You wouldn't believe how many times I've replayed that Christmas Day scenario in my head, longing to go back and choose a different present. A set of hair straighteners, a new iPhone or vouchers for her favourite clothes shop. Anything but those tickets. I'm sure I'm not the only person or fan who thinks that. But hindsight is a wonderful thing.

I kept the T-shirt on for the rest of the day. 'As Ariana's boyfriend, I have to be the one who takes you,' I said. We'd already been to see JLS a few times and Little Mix. Concerts were our dad and daughter thing.

But I hadn't counted on Bad/Sad Martin becoming so powerful. In *Superman III*, Bad Superman does mean things like straighten the leaning tower of Pisa and blow out the Olympic Torch (I know, I can laugh at it now), progressing to more serious acts like detonating an oil tanker. Overriding everything was his hatred of, and determination to kill, Clark Kent, or Good Superman. The same battle was raging inside my head. January is a grim month at the best of times. But as each dark morning dawned Bad/Sad Martin was pulling me further and further into the depths of despair and self-loathing. In the motivational talks I now give, I liken him to a 'dementor', a creature from the *Harry Potter* world – sucking every ounce of happiness and positivity from your body. 'You'll have no sense of self any more … no anything … you'll just exist. As an empy shell,' describes one character. And that's it, right there. That's depression. It's like being trapped in a goldfish bowl. All around you, the world carries on turning; you watch as people live their lives, laugh, joke and smile. But a thick glass barrier separates you from them. You'll never join them again. Ever.

By February, I was in freefall. Manchester United were playing Southampton in the EFL (English Football League) cup final at Wembley. 'What do you mean you're not going?' Gabby quizzed me.

'I can't,' I mumbled. 'I've got Eve.'

She stared at me incredulously. I could have arranged for Eve to stay with her mum, my mum or Gabby. But Bad/Sad Martin had done a good job convincing me that I didn't deserve to go. Didn't deserve to be a part of it. This swirling, spreading, blackness inside me was twisting and tainting everything... my mind, my thoughts, my convictions.

The fan I sold my tickets to couldn't believe his luck. 'Why are you not going, mate?' he asked.

'Oh, you know, childcare,' I said, nonchalantly. 'It's just one of those things. There'll be other games.'

I parroted the same answers to everyone who asked. Mike, my brothers, my colleagues. The more I acted upon Bad/Sad Martin's suggestions, the more powerful he became. Soon, I decided, there'd be no more games. No more cuddles with Eve and Gabby. No more dog walks. It sounds unbelievable now but I honestly didn't think about the impact taking my own life would have on my loved ones. I say 'loved ones' but, in my sick mind, it was a case of me loving them. That love wasn't returned. They'd be glad to see the back of me. I'd be doing them a favour. As I say in my motivational talks, I'm horrified that I came so close to putting Eve, Gabby, my mum, even Alfie through such an ordeal. But depression does that. Bad/Sad Martin's taunts and jeers were hitting the bullseye every single time. I believed every single word. With my mind made up, that streak of Hibbert stubbornness came into its own. If I'm going to do something, I do it well. There'd be no coming back from this. I chose the time and place. A Friday afternoon in early February.

As the countdown began, I felt resigned to my fate; partly numb but also relieved that I wouldn't have to pretend any more. This pain would finally be over. Not long now. On the Wednesday evening, I dug out one of my favourite photos. It was of me on my stag night, just three years earlier, surrounded by my friends. I gazed at the image and felt a pang of envy for happy-go-lucky Martin smiling for the camera. It was like looking at a different person. I clicked on 'forward' then typed three words 'I love you' and sent it to Mum, Danny and Andy.

I've never shared these details with anyone before. Reading this chapter, Gabby was upset that I hadn't sent her the picture and message too. 'I had something else for you,' I confessed. Thankfully, I never needed to send it. On the Thursday morning at work, on what I'd planned to be my penultimate day on this Earth, my phone beeped. It was a message from Danny. As the words registered, my stomach lurched and a wave of nausea washed over me. Gripping my desk, I lowered myself into my chair, wiped the prickle of sweat from my upper lip and read it again.

The message was clearly intended for Mum. But, by mistake, Danny had sent it to me. There it was, in black-and-white. 'Mum, do you think Martin's going to commit suicide?' My heart thumped in my chest. Adrenalin surged through every vein. My bowels turned to water.

Shit. Shit shit shit. I'd been found out.

Bad/Sad Martin was furious. *Bloody, interfering, *^*%$. Why can't people stop interfering and leave us alone?*

But the real Martin had just been given a violent wake-up call. That message was the equivalent of a swift, sharp, slap across the face. A bucket of ice-cold water being emptied over my head. Being grabbed by the lapels and shaken like a rag doll until my teeth rattled. I felt like a sleepwalker waking up to find they were on the brink of stepping in front of a train or off a cliff edge. So close. So bloody close. My chest heaved. I gasped for breath.

With trembling hands, I managed to type a response. 'Don't be stupid, Danny.' Shakily, I exhaled. Tried to calm my breathing. I was sure of one thing. I needed help. And I needed it now. Picking up the phone, I rang my boss. 'I'm not well,' I said. 'I need to take some time off.' Next, I rang my GP surgery and managed to get an appointment that same afternoon. My GP asked me to fill in a mental health questionnaire. It asked me all the usual questions. 'Have you found little pleasure or interest in doing things? Have you thought about harming yourself? Trouble sleeping? Feeling angry?' My pen flew over the page. Tick. Tick. Tick.

Wordlessly, I handed it back. She quickly scanned my answers. 'OK, you've got the top score which means alarm bells are ringing,' she said gently. 'However, there's a six-month waiting list for counselling.'

I stared at her blankly. How could I tell her I wouldn't be here then? With a reassuring smile, she made the referral and said I'd be informed when an appointment was available.

Back at home, I knew I couldn't wait. Googling treatments for depression I came across a type of psychotherapy called 'Eye Movement Desensitisation and Reprocessing' (EMDR). It wasn't well-known in the UK but in the US was used as a way of treating troops suffering from PTSD (post-traumatic stress disorder). It also had great results for treating depression and anxiety.

Even better, there was a qualified practitioner half an hour's drive away. It was a hundred pounds a session, money I didn't have. But Mum, bless her, helped me out when I told her how bad things had become. She and Gabby were the only ones I confided in. Bizarrely, my brother and I have never spoken of that text he sent. It was simply never mentioned. He has no idea that that slip of the finger when he sent it to me instead of Mum saved my life. I'm still trying to find the right time to have that conversation and thank him. Because, thanks to my brother's intervention, on the day I should have been ending my life, I was taking the first steps to ensuring I stayed very much alive.

This is my layman's take on how EMDR works. When you experience trauma, your body protects you. It puts it in a box and closes the lid. However, the trauma, the upset, that hasn't been processed, doesn't stay buried. It seeps, leaches into your subconscious. Traditional counselling wouldn't have worked for me. It's reliant upon opening up. If you don't talk, the counsellor can't help you. Sometimes, as in my case, we don't even know what's caused the trauma or negative emotion in the first place. EMDR is about safely opening the box in your brain containing the things that upset you and processing your way through them. Its therapists have different methods to bilaterally stimulate the brain and open up the memory box; mine got me to hold onto two prongs. They would vibrate in turn, the left, followed by the right. I'd then close my eyes and move my eyes to the left, then right, matching the vibrations. Then I'd reveal what was coming to mind.

Among the traumas she identified were Mum and Dad's divorce, Granddad's death, the breakdown of my relationship with Sarah and the separation from Eve.

'But Mum and Dad got divorced when I was nineteen,' I argued. 'And Grandad died thirteen years ago.'

However, it doesn't matter how long ago these things happened or how insignificant they might have felt at the time. They'd caused hurt. Hurt that had never healed. EMDR doesn't involve talking about trauma in detail, but processing and storing it in a different, non-hurting, way. In those eight weeks, I learned so much about the structures of my own depression; what it was and what it fed off. It helped me make sense of my feelings and how to manage them. It was like peeling off the layers of an onion. Crucially, the therapist also helped me identify a 'happy place' in my mind where I could retreat.

That was easy. Our honeymoon: St Lucia with Gabby. Whenever I need to, I close my eyes and I'm there, walking hand-in-hand along the beach with my wife. I can feel the soft, white sand, marvel at the azure sea lapping at my feet, sense the warm sun on my face, giving me strength.

I left each session that little less sad, that bit more hopeful. Bad/Sad Martin was losing his powers. The real me was getting stronger. Halfway through the eight-week course, I felt strong enough to hand my notice in permanently. I was going to set up my own sporting agency, recruiting footballers for teams. At the end of the final session, in April 2017, I walked out of that room with my head held high. I felt like me again. I drove home listening to Ariana Grande music.

Walking Alfie in the woods, I would stop for no reason. I'd look around and breathe in fresh, spring air. I'd stare, entranced, at the carpets of crocuses, stop and listen to the birds singing in the branches above – I used to moan when birds woke me up singing in the summer! – the crack of twigs underfoot. I felt like Dorothy marvelling at the colourful land of Oz. I knew I wasn't magically cured. I would always have depression. Bad/Sad/Sick Martin would always be there. But I understood him now and what made him tick. I could talk to him, assure him, reason with him, distract him, calm him. Manage him. More than anything, I'd realised I was blessed. I had a beautiful daughter, a wife, family and friends who did love me. I could see that now. Life was a precious gift. And I was going to live it to the full.

Exactly four weeks later, I was blown up by a suicide bomber.

5

22 May 2017

In the run-up to the concert I was a new man. I was sleeping soundly, eating healthily, taking Alfie for long romps through the woods. My therapy had made me re-evaluate so many things. I'd decided not to return to banking and instead focus full time on my agency, Synergy Sports Management. I already had some good players and team managers on my books. And I was listening to Ariana Grande continuously, on Eve's orders, so I'd know some of the songs on the night. Eve and I would play them loudly in the car over our weekends together.

The concert was on a Monday night. With Eve about to enter year ten – when she'd start studying for her GCSEs – I promised not to have her home too late. She'd set her heart on being a vet and knew she'd have to work especially hard to get good grades.

I drove to Mum's from Bradford as soon as I'd finished meetings that day. I was going to stay over after the concert and drop Eve at school. I'd kissed Gabby goodbye that morning as she headed off for work. 'See you tomorrow,' I'd said. It was a glorious day. SUMMER IS FINALLY HERE, trumpeted the weather reports.

Eve wore black jeans, a black vest and black cardigan and her freshly washed, shoulder-length hair was glossy. 'You look lovely,' I told her, giving her a hug. 'Ready to see me do some dad dancing?' I chortled. I'd decided against the 'Ariana Grande is my Girlfriend' T-shirt and wore jeans, a shirt and navy jumper. With Ariana playing full blast, we'd driven into Manchester city centre for a pre-concert meal at our favourite Italian restaurant, San Carlo.

The waiter poured water into Eve's wineglass and she sipped it delicately. 'Cheers,' I said, clinking my fruit juice against her glass. 'Here's to a great night.'

My beautiful daughter chattered away as she tucked into her pizza, telling me all about her day at school. Her eyes twinkled under the soft lighting and I was, suddenly, struck by how grown-up she was getting. She was wearing a smidgeon of mascara and lip gloss. She'd started carrying a handbag. In a few short years, she'd be sipping wine for real. 'So, this is when it starts,' I ventured.

She frowned. 'When what starts?'

'Oh, you know,' I said. 'The knocks on the door.' She stared at me quizzically. 'From admiring young men.'

She blushed furiously and laughed self-consciously. 'Stop it, Daddy.'

But I couldn't wipe this daft grin off my face. My daughter was turning into a beautiful young woman with the world at her feet. She had friends who loved her, was doing well at school and was a joy to be around. In that moment, I'd never felt closer to her. I couldn't believe that in four months she'd be fifteen. How had that happened? She would always be my little girl but I could already see she was blossoming into a young woman. I wanted our closeness to continue and for her to be able to talk to me about anything and everything.

Friends had been talking about their daughters dating, bringing boyfriends home to meet the family. Part of me was dreading the prospect. I prayed she'd meet someone wonderful. A United fan? I could take him to the football matches with me. I imagined me walking her proudly up the aisle, giving my 'father of the bride' speech. Holding my first grandchild in my arms. As a waiter went past, I stopped him. 'Could you take a photo of me with my daughter, please?' I asked. He stood to my left and captured the moment beautifully. Me beaming proudly, Eve smiling shyly with her lips clamped together. We're both holding our glasses in the air.

I never posted pictures of Eve on social media but I was so proud in that moment that I uploaded it to my Twitter page. 'Quick pit stop with Eve @SanCarlo_Group #Manchester before a date with @ArianaGrande', I typed. The time was 6.53 p.m. In the time to come that photo would appear on news pages and TV screens around the world: 'Just hours from disaster.'

Our VIP tickets included free parking at the AO Arena multi-storey car park. I chose a spot close to the exit so we could make a speedy getaway among the fourteen thousand concert-goers. Served by just one main road, you can be caught in snarling post-concert traffic for hours. 'We'll need to leave before the encore to beat the traffic,' I told Eve. 'You've got school tomorrow.'

She nodded. 'That's fine, Daddy,' she said.

We walked across the City Room – an open lobby which leads from the car park and Victoria train station to the arena. It's one of three entrances serving the arena – one of those big, airy spaces that you don't give too much thought to as you hurry through. It's just there. As we passed the merchandise stalls, I sensed her slowing. Yep, she was gazing at the official tour hoodies. I grinned. 'Go on, then. My treat,' I said.

'Really?' she exclaimed. 'Thanks, Daddy.' She took her time: black, white or pink? Hood or no hood? Eventually, she settled on a black hoodie with an image of the singer and 'Dangerous Woman' logo emblazoned across the front. On the back was a list of tour performances. 'There's Manchester!' she cried, pointing to the words. I handed over forty pounds and Eve insisted on pulling the top over her cardigan despite the heat of the night.

'Lovely,' I said admiringly. Eve looked longingly at the glossy programme but I baulked at the ten-pound price tag.

Our seats, in the front row of box number four, were fantastic. Situated above the lower tiers, they gave us a fantastic view of the stage down below and to our left. 'This is amazing,' Eve breathed, leaning on the barrier to gaze at the seats below. Below us, thousands of teenage girls thronged excitedly. Eve couldn't get her head around the fact that the VIP tickets meant free drinks and snacks all night. 'What, so I can just go and get a coke and won't have to pay?' she asked. I nodded. 'Whenever I want? Could I get three if I wanted to?'

Back she came, clutching two glasses – one for each of us. 'You were right, Daddy,' she said, delighted. 'They were free. This is *brilliant*.'

Two artists, Victoria Monét and Bia, performed first. A giant projection of a digital clock counted down from thirty minutes, twenty minutes, ten minutes. The excitement and anticipation started to build. Then there were twenty seconds, ten seconds, five seconds... I've attended cup finals and tournaments all over the world. But nothing, *nothing*, could have prepared me for the noise of 14,000 teenage girls, all screaming at the top of their lungs, as their heroine appeared on stage. Eve laughed as I clamped my hands over my ears, grimacing dramatically. *Bloody hell*. I imagined every glass, window or mirror within a three-mile radius spontaneously shattering.

Wearing her hair in her trademark high ponytail and impossibly high boots, the star – surrounded by buff, muscled dancers in black sleeveless tops – put on one heck of a show. Her incredible, pitch-perfect voice soared to the very rafters of the arena. She performed intricate choreographed routines without even breaking a sweat.

For the next ninety minutes we were entertained. We were entranced. We were enthralled. We belted out all her hits, we bopped to the fast songs and waved our arms aloft during the ballads. At one point, I stood behind Eve and took her hands in mine, swaying her playfully from side to side. If she was embarrassed by my dad dancing, she didn't show it.

'She's brilliant,' I leaned down to shout in Eve's ear. 'You'd swear she was miming to a CD.' We both held up our phones, capturing songs and performances. I forwarded some to Gabby. 'Amazing night,' I wrote.

Costume changes were swift, dramatic and effortless: a little black dress with pearls; baggy, white cargo pants and crop top; orange jumpsuit. Ariana is one of those people who could wear a bin bag and still look amazing. I remember smiling at my daughter's beautiful face lit up by the spotlights and lasers as she danced and sang along. She knew every single word to every single song.

After a rendition of one of her most well-known hits, 'One Last Time', the star left the stage to prepare for the encore. Eve saw me glance at my watch. 'We need to go, don't we?' she said with a sad smile. Ariana was finishing with 'Dangerous Woman', the album's title song. As I nodded, my lovely girl didn't roll her eyes or say it wasn't fair. She simply reached for my outstretched hand and, giving a backward glance over her shoulder, as if to capture every last moment to memory, she followed me out. We chattered and clattered all the way down the largely empty steps to the outside corridors. Out of the arena, the lighting was stark and bright. A few other sensible souls like us were making an early escape before the crowds.

In the distance, we could hear the screams and stamping of feet greeting Ariana as she reappeared on stage. 'We'll watch it on YouTube,' I said and she squeezed my hand in response. Retracing our steps back towards the car, we reached the doors which led back into the City Room. The nondescript room. The throughfare.

If you imagine looking at it from above, concert-leavers heading to the car park or train station would cross this space from west to east. At the moment, there was a trickle of people. Within minutes it would become a fast-flowing river – all pouring through the doors, keen to get home, dreaming of a hot cuppa.

As the arena doors swung closed behind us, the sound of Ariana's singing became muffled.

Around a hundred parents milled about, waiting patiently for their teenage kids to emerge, flushed and exuberant, from the show. Like me, most had probably bought the tickets for birthdays or Christmas. They had congratulated themselves for a great gift choice, smiled indulgently as their kids counted down the days on the calendar, planned what to wear. No doubt, for many, it was the first time they'd let their teenagers go to a venue without an adult. With a pang, I realised it was just a matter of time before Eve announced that she'd like to attend her next concert with her friends rather than her old dad. I'd be the one waiting in the lobby for her, glancing at my phone screen, jangling my car keys.

These smiling, tired-looking, devoted parents had one eye on the arena doors, one eye on their phone screens... checking for messages or tapping quick texts. 'Am here. Try not to be long – you've got school tomorrow.' Finishing with an 'X' for a kiss or a fond emoji. Eve was in the middle of exams preparing her for GCSEs. Others would have been sitting the real thing, but enjoying a rare night off from their revision.

As the doors opened and closed behind us, more frequently, Ariana's voice came and went like a tide. I imagined the final roar of appreciation, the lights coming up. Everyone gathering their bags, heading for the exit. Instinctively, I picked up my pace. Ahead of us rose two flights of stairs which led up to the mezzanine. To the left was JD Williams, the fashion store. To the right, a McDonald's. To the right and left of these stairs were the doors leading to the car park. We were heading for the right-hand side. I have no memory of walking past a young man with a large rucksack on his back.

Although I remember very little of what happened next, I imagine Eve calling out 'Daddy, Daddy, slow down,' as I trotted on ahead, forgetting her legs were shorter than mine.

'Sorry, love, you go ahead,' I'd have said, ushering her ahead of me and falling in behind her. It was a move which saved her life.

I kept my eye on the car park door. We were halfway across the room. A few steps further on and then—

BOOM!

For a few seconds, there was nothing but noise. A high-pitched, deafening noise. It roared through my ears and surged inside my brain. I felt my feet leave the ground. I was in the air. I was underwater. Just ahead of me, the steps shook, juddered then turned onto their side. It took a few seconds for me to realise that I was lying on the ground, dazed and winded.

What the—

Instinctively, I tried to move but nothing happened. I shook my head in confusion trying to get my thoughts to settle. The loud initial bang had stopped but inside my head it was reverberating like an echo. Through the jumble of possibilities – runaway truck, car, train, one word flashed inside my head. 'Bomb'. That's all it could be. We all know now, of course, that the man we had hurried past a few seconds earlier was suicide bomber Salman Abedi. His heavy rucksack – causing him to stoop – contained more than three thousand nuts and bolts packed tightly around a homemade explosive device. Individually, these small bits of metal are harmless enough. But blasted through the air at speed they become deadly weapons. They left golf-ball-sized holes in concrete walls and metal doors. So you can only imagine what they did to human flesh.

Eve. EVE!

For a second, I raised my head an inch off the ground before it sank, heavily, back into position. *Where is she?* I was lying on my right side, my head pillowed against my outstretched arm. The City Room was unrecognisable. The stark whiteness of the ceiling and walls was gone. It was now grey, smoky, acrid. My hearing was muffled, as if I was being held six feet underwater. But it felt eerily silent. As my lips parted, then closed, I grimaced at the metallic tang hitting my taste buds. Blood. I felt it filling my mouth, gargling and bubbling in my throat and chest. I tried to cough to clear it. Nothing happened. *Can't breathe...*

Beneath me, the ground felt cold and hard. Rock hard. Suddenly, my nostrils twitched. Neurons fired to and from my brain, trying to make sense of the smell, the stench, now filling my nasal passages. Fire, acrid, shocking smoke, burned clothes, singed hair, charred flesh, hot tar. Nausea stirred the depths of my stomach as it dawned on me. Death. It was the smell of death.

I blinked once, twice, three times, trying to control the urge to vomit. My eyes were now taking in scenes of horror unfolding all around me in slow motion, before settling on Eve. She was just a few metres ahead of me. Just out of reach. Lying on her front, on her left cheek. Her eyes were closed. Blood trickled from her gaping mouth as she gasped for breath. The area around her right temple had been ripped open. The gaping hole exposed brain tissue. I tried to call her name but made just a desperate croak.

Dear God. I needed to reach her. Instinctively, I tried to move – but nothing happened. It felt like I'd been encased in quick-setting cement. A growing sense of panic took hold. Stay calm, stay calm, I urged myself. I tried again. 'Eve?' I croaked. There was no response, no flicker of recognition. No turning of her head towards the sound of my voice.

'You're OK,' I gasped. 'I'm here. Daddy's here.' She continued to gasp. Like a fish out of water.

Help. Please help us.

My desperate gaze landed on an object a few feet away. An arm. On its own.

Was it mine? Summoning all my energy, I looked up to my right then down to my left. There were my arms, my fingers, wiggling weakly back at me. Thank God. My upper limbs were still intact.

Next, my eyes roamed down my denim-clad legs, towards my feet. My jumper and jeans were covered in holes. But my legs and feet were still there, encased in my brand-new Hugo Boss shoes and stripey, multi-coloured Paul Smith socks. I was intact. That was something.

If this was a Hollywood film, there would have been alarms blaring, cries for help, survivors scrambling to their feet, bystanders running for help, as the dust settled. But here, in real life, it was eerily quiet. Afterwards, I discovered why. Most of those in the blast zone had died instantly. Others, like Eve, had sustained such horrific injuries they were unable to make a sound. Behind me, I could hear moans and whimpers from the few who had survived and were still conscious. I sensed movement, as a few began to stagger or crawl to safety.

I became aware of a growing sense of clammy wetness seeping through the front of my body – soaking into my clothes. Had I landed in a puddle? A spilt drink? And then the colour registered. It was my blood, creeping across the cold, tiled, marble-effect floor. The speckled pattern on the tiles were gradually disappearing as it spread like a silent cloak. It was coming out from beneath me and out of my left arm, draped in front of me. *This is bad.*

I'd been blasted by twenty-two pieces of deadly shrapnel. One had lodged itself in my spine. Another had ruptured a major artery in my neck, causing massive blood loss.

A cold, calm thought resonated through the confusion: *I'm dying.* I had one job to do before I went. That was to get Eve out. Now, there were footsteps and voices. A flash of a high-vis jacket. A crackle of radio. Shoes appeared in front of me. Someone was crouching down. Then hands reached under my head. Something soft was pressed firmly into my neck. 'You OK there?' a male voice asked.

'Eve,' I whispered. 'My daughter.' I was staring intently at her, willing my saviour to leave me – and help her. But he either didn't hear me or didn't understand. From behind, a woman's voice was barking instructions. Something about continuing to apply pressure. Keeping him – me – conscious. The sensation of pushing into my neck intensified. 'You're OK,' the voice assured me. 'Help is on its way.'

The pool of crimson liquid – made up of two separate rivers gushing from my body – was growing all the time. While staring at Eve, trying not to blink, I could see the blood out of the corner of my eye creeping insidiously, closer and closer to my mouth. Instinctively, I tried to move my head away but this disturbed my view of Eve. I stayed put.

The voice, in a strong Mancunian accent, kept up a continual stream of chatter. 'What's your name? Where do you live? Who do you support?' His voice was strong, calm and reassuring. It took all my effort to gasp each one-word answer. Still the questions came. 'How was the concert? Ariana Grande – was she good? She sounded good.' I closed my eyes, silently willing him to stop talking. This wasn't the time for chit-chat. 'Martin?' he persisted. 'Martin?'

I whimpered. 'Please,' I whispered, trying to gesture towards her with my eyes. 'My daughter.'

'How old are you, Martin?'

I grimaced and tried again. He wasn't listening. 'Help Eve,' I gasped. '*Help. My. Daughter.*' Frustration welled up. Why was no one else running in to help? 'Where are the ambulances?' I panted weakly. In fact, where were the emergency services – full stop?

'They're on their way,' the voice assured me.

A sense of wooziness was washing over me. The blood was an inch from my open mouth. Now a centimetre. Now a millimetre. And there it was, a warm wetness against my lips. My own blood nuzzling my mouth. A movement caught my eye and turned what little blood there was left in my veins to ice. I can't see her. *I can't see Eve.* I could see her hoodie, her jeans, her trainers. But someone had placed a white covering over her head. *They think she's dead.*

Every fibre, every cell, in my body protested. Terror, panic and fear swelled within me. I imagined poor Eve – desperately trying to take in oxygen underneath the covering. I needed to yell, to roar, to rise to my feet, snatch the snowy-white, shroud-like, covering away and demand that someone treat her, save her. But nothing happened. I was the only person who could help her, who knew she was still alive. But I was trapped in a dying body. From deep within, a furious strength erupted. It rose up through my oesophagus and out through my mouth, resulting in a guttural noise. 'Nnnngggg,' I gasped to get my helper's attention. 'She's alive, she's breathing,' I panted, staring intently at the covered body of my daughter. Nothing happened. No one had heard me. I tried again. Louder this time. 'She's ALIVE!' The effort drained me. Another flurried movement and the covering was pulled back. I could see Eve's beautiful, torn, face once more.

Her breathing was shallower now. Her lips quivered with the effort of staying alive. 'Stay,' I gasped, praying she could hear me. 'Stay with me, Eve. I'm here.'

Time crawled by. In the distance, I could hear sirens. Thank God, I thought, waiting for the cavalry to burst in. And waited. 'Where the hell *are* they?' I heard someone snap in despair. *My thoughts exactly.*

My eyes stung with the effort of staring at Eve but I couldn't let up for a second. Suddenly, there was another flurry near her. Once again, she disappeared from view. Once again, I was consumed by rage and grunted my protests. *For the love of God, stop covering her. She's alive!*

From all directions of the room, mobile phones rang out forlornly and went unanswered. People called to each other. There was a rattling of metal, fabric being ripped, boxes being unclipped, packets torn open.

'They'll be here soon,' my rescuer assured me. I shook my head. I'd never felt so alone, so abandoned. 'You. Said. That. Ages. Ago,' I hissed angrily through clenched teeth and gasps. The effort of speaking exhausted me. It was taking all my effort to breathe. I was tired. So very tired. After each blissful blink, it took colossal energy to force open my eyelids again. I had to stay conscious for

Eve. What if someone covered her up yet again? I was the only one who could save her. My eyes felt gritty, then twitched with the effort of keeping them trained on her. I started to shiver uncontrollably.

I stirred, sensing hands beneath me. My head was lifted clear of the pool of blood. My cheek felt wet and cold. I shivered again. 'Martin?' said my saviour. 'We're going to take you outside to the ambulances. Hold tight.'

Eve was still lying, ignored and alone, on the ground. I tried to wriggle. I scrunched up my face with effort, shook my head and forced the sound out again – louder. A face loomed. 'Take Eve. Please, save my daughter,' I begged.

Words were exchanged above me then, thank God, I was back on the wet floor. My cheek was immersed once more in my growing pool of blood. Through drooping eyelids, like a curtain lowering on a darkened stage, I watched Eve being scooped onto a piece of hoarding from a merchandise stand and carried away. 'Thank you,' I whispered. 'Thank you.' By now, I was shaking uncontrollably and my teeth chattered loudly. Relief surged through my veins. 'Eve is safe,' a voice said in my head. 'She'll be OK. You can go now.' For a moment, I almost smiled. 'Only you, Martin,' I chided myself, 'of all the places to go, on the bloody floor of an arena.' I felt a sudden pang of sadness at never seeing Eve, Gabby, Alfie, my mum, my brothers ever again. I longed to reach out to them. To tell them how much I loved them. I would miss them.

My saviour was leaning over me. 'Tell my wife,' I gasped, 'please. Tell Gabby I love her.' Even now, six years on, thinking of those moments, that conviction that I'd never see her face again, brings hot tears. I allowed myself to sink deeper into the floor. It was no longer cold and hard but warm, soft and welcoming. My breathing was slowing now. Slower still. 'Martin?' my saviour called. 'Martin?' His voice should have been getting louder but it was drifting further and further away from me. A soft, snowy whiteness engulfed me like a feather-filled duvet, bringing with it a sense of peace and calm. There was no fear or pain. Just relief. Blessed relief.

I was going.

I was gone.

6

The Aftermath

'Martin…'

  '*Mar*tin…'

Cogs slowly shifted, turned and clicked inside my brain. The voice sounded far away.

  '*MAR*tin.'

Something fired inside my brain – like a pilot light flaring on a boiler – triggering a flicker of recognition. Karl? My Liverpool-supporting friend from banking. My eyelids fluttered. 'Hey Martin,' said the voice, delighted at getting a response. There was a silhouette sitting by my bed. His face came into focus. Yep, it was Karl. I grimaced, trying to make sense of all the jumbled thoughts whirling around my head. 'Hey, guess what?' he said, eyes twinkling. 'You've got no pants on under that sheet. All the nurses have been in to have a right good laugh at your knob.'

From deep inside, a bubble of laughter started to form, swell and rise up inside me. But as my diaphragm expanded to provide my body with extra air, I froze. Lay rigid. Every cell, every fibre of my being, was on fire. Excruciating pain fizzed through my veins, spreading through my body. It was as if fireworks were going off. I cried out but the pain only increased. Now I was coughing… *Bloody hell. I can't breathe.*

Finally, I was lying still. Panting, aware of tubes up my nose and coming out of my body in all directions. When the pain had eased, I shook my head and frowned. I hoped he could understand me. *Don't make me laugh, Karl. For the love of God, don't make me laugh.*

I remember very little of the weeks following 22 May 2017. It's all a technicolour blur with just a few very lucid, random, moments. That was one of them. Just thinking about his comment makes me laugh. Karl and I spend all our time ribbing both each other – and our rival football teams. The first half hour of any phone call or meeting is spent hurling ever-more outrageous insults at each other.

Otherwise, there's a huge blank in my brain in those early weeks after the bombing. Gabby did video some of my recovery but I have to brace myself to watch those recordings. I imagine it's like watching footage of yourself enthusiastically leading the 'Macarena' after one too many – only just not quite as entertaining. Even seven years on, it triggers feelings of sadness and anxiety. No matter how hard I rack my brains, the memories just aren't there. So, writing these next couple of chapters has involved long detailed chats with those who were.

Hearing accounts from the paramedic and surgeon who saved my life, the major trauma nurse and physiotherapist who enabled me to start living again, the local resident who ran towards the arena and spent hours tending to the dying and wounded, has been humbling, astounding, shocking and hard to believe. Before that night they were complete strangers. Today, I am honoured and privileged to call them my friends. I will never, ever be able to fully repay them for what they did.

And then there's the stark reality of hearing the impact of the atrocity on my loved ones... The unfolding horror of knowing that Eve and I had been caught up in the bombing – with no idea if we were dead or alive – must have been horrendous for them. So many thousands of people must have been worried sick that night, in the depths of despair as they made phone calls. Most of them, thankfully, got the news they wanted – their loved one was alive, albeit with injuries and scars – both physical and emotional. For so many other people who lost a loved one that night, that pain has never eased. They've simply grown used to living with it.

I'll start by going back to the moment of 10.31 p.m. in the City Room, the moment twenty-two-year-old terrorist Salman Abedi detonated his home-made bomb. As Eve and I had been walking from west to east across the City Room, we'd passed him standing motionless in the middle of the space. He'd been a conspicuous figure, almost doubled over from the immense weight of his plus-30-kg, or five-and-a-half stone, rucksack containing the crude explosive device he'd assembled in his Manchester flat. In the formal inquiry into the atrocity which began three years later, we learned that some parents waiting to pick up their children had already expressed concerns about him. But I have no recollection of seeing him. I was focused on the car park doors ahead. Getting out and hitting the road before everyone else. Eve and I were hand-in-hand, she was fractionally ahead of me.

We were six metres away when he detonated his bomb. He was completely obliterated in the blast. Those poor souls – innocent kids, loving parents – within a five-metre radius around him didn't have a chance. Eve and I were the closest survivors. Others who died were further away from us.

The blast tore mobile phones and wallets out of hands and pockets, causing huge identification problems in those early few hours. Other than me gasping 'Martin' to the security guard when he asked me my name, no one had the faintest idea who I was.

'Martin' is a name that Paul Harvey – the brilliant paramedic assigned to take me to hospital that night – could never forget. He must have shouted it hundreds of times in a desperate bid to keep me conscious while I was in his ambulance. The fact I'm even here to tell my story is thanks to him.

A couple of hours into his night shift, he had just dropped a patient off at Manchester Royal Infirmary when messages started coming over the radio. 'There were initial reports of an explosion; then a fire,' he recalls. Ambulances were summoned to a rendezvous point but frustratingly, appallingly, tragically weren't allowed into the arena immediately to treat those who so badly needed emergency help.

Paul was initially assigned to help with the walking wounded. He remembers one distraught teenage girl with her hands clamped to the sides of her head. The blast had perforated her eardrums, leaving her unable to hear a sound. There were also victims clearly suffering from shock and trauma; lone, weeping, frightened teenagers separated from friends, distraught families trying to find missing loved ones. The whole scene was horrific. Finally, he was summoned to the clearing area set up on a platform of Victoria Station for seriously injured casualties who had been carried out of the arena on advertising hoardings. Paul remembers being told 'the next patient is ready for moving'.

'You were in a bad way, Martin,' he recalls now. 'You were pale and clammy and vomiting blood as a result of internal bleeding.' This occurs when the blood has nowhere else left to go. Paramedics explained I'd lost a lot of blood and they had started to administer intravenous fluids. 'Your clinical observations were quite shocking. You were showing signs of hypovolemia, or clinical shock, due to loss of blood volume and you also had reduced levels of consciousness.'

Paul and his colleague got me onto their stretcher and into their ambulance and prepared me for the journey. Then a manager appeared at the back doors and said 'This one's for Wythenshawe Hospital.' As Paul explains now, he was clearly trying to divide casualties between the area's hospitals. But Paul was having none of it. I have no doubt whatsoever that his response, his conviction in that moment that that wasn't the right decision and his courage in saying so, saved my life. In no uncertain times he told the manager that I wouldn't make it. I was critically injured and speed was of the essence. He insisted I needed to go to Salford Royal Infirmary instead. It was closer – just 4.4 miles away – I'd be seen quicker and I had a better chance of surviving. After a 'heated discussion', the manager agreed I could be taken to Salford instead.

Now, Paul was a longstanding and experienced paramedic and I thank God he was allocated to treat me that night. A newly qualified, less gutsy, less feisty paramedic might have followed orders to the letter. Taken me to Wythenshawe which was nine miles away, south of the city. Paul has no doubt I'd have died en route. I think it's partly for this reason I have such affection for Salford Royal. I see it as a beacon of hope shining brightly for me on that dark night.

Paul remembers me, between episodes of bringing up blood, asking about Eve. Where is she? How is she? Did she get out? 'One of the things I've learned in more than twenty years of being a paramedic is to never lie to patients,' he tells me. 'So, I'd never say, "She's fine." I'd have said, "Somebody else will be looking after her and she will be getting the best treatment possible." And you seemed reassured by that.'

A medical team was on standby and rushed me straight into the resuscitation room. 'After a quick handover to the doctors on the team, that was it,' Paul recalls. 'I can remember walking out of the resus room with the trolley. And there was chaos... other crews turning up, people looking for relatives. It was really distressing. Part of the job is that everything hits you afterwards.'

At some point in the early hours, I was transferred to intensive care and put under the care of neurosurgeon Mr Ankur Saxena, who had arrived early for his day shift after being alerted to a major incident. His biggest concern was the rupture of the carotid artery on the right side of my neck which was potentially life-threatening, as it can cause a stroke. 'It sounds horrible now but we kind of accepted that you were going to be paralysed,' he says now. 'The whole focus was to save your life.' There was no way of 'treating' the ruptured artery or another which had been 'nicked' by the impact of the bolt hitting. 'We just had to make sure it didn't continue to bleed massively.' From then on it was a case of observing me closely and carrying out investigations to see the impact of the rupture.

'There was no blood flow to the brain through the artery on that side. But the brain is supplied via multiple arteries, which all form a network. And they "kicked in" as a result of the artery rupturing. We call it collateral circulation. This only happens in younger patients. Whether the blood supply is good enough or not is variable. In your case, clearly it was. However, there will always be a greater risk of stroke. We decided to continue to monitor you before operating on your shrapnel wounds and spine. It was a calculated risk but we agreed on forty-eight to seventy-two hours.'

The bolt that tore through my neck at high speed should have exited on the other side of my neck – virtually decapitating me. It didn't. This is what I've surmised from many conversations with medics over the years. By some freak, million-to-one chance, I'd gulped at the precise moment the bolt was travelling through my neck. In that split second, I'd swallowed the shrapnel. Instead of continuing its deadly journey, tearing through my neck and throat, it had meandered down my oesophagus and ended up in my stomach, where it was recovered during surgery.

'It must have gone down like a pinball! How did you do that?' Gabby asked incredulously when I was writing this chapter.

'Er, I don't think I had a choice in the matter, love,' I told her, equally incredulous at her question.

However, she's always maintained I have a gift in being able to swallow a tablet without the need for water. Whereas she can down a pint and a paracetamol will still be sitting stubbornly on her tongue! Or maybe my great-grandmother or a higher power was watching over Eve and me that night and ensured I swallowed the nut rather than allowing it to complete its deadly journey through my neck.

My family were given a bleak prognosis when they finally tracked me down, although very little sank in to begin with. Andy, my youngest brother, had been the first to know something was amiss. He'd just arrived home from his Monday night tennis session when a breaking news item flashed up on his phone. *Reports of an incident at the Manchester Arena.* 'Oh God,' he'd said to his wife, Kelly. 'Martin and Eve are there.' He'd immediately called Mum who was watching a TV show and blissfully ignorant. 'Have you heard?' he asked. 'Something's happened at the arena.' He said he'd try to reach us but was sure it was nothing to worry about. His wife, Kelly, rang Eve while he rang me. One line rang out. The other was dead.

'I'll ring Gabby,' Mum told him. 'Maybe she's in contact with him.'

Sleepily (she and Alfie had gone to bed early), Gabby had confirmed that, yes, she had heard from me. 'He sent me a couple of messages and videos from the concert,' she'd said.

'But other than that?' Mum pushed.

'No.'

When Mum explained something had happened at the arena and no one could reach either me or Eve, Gabby didn't bat an eyelid. 'Oh, his battery will have gone 'cos of all the videos he took. Don't worry, I'm sure it's nothing. It'll be fine.' She was used to my phone running out of juice at the most inconvenient times and my tardiness in remembering to recharge it. But after ringing off, Gabby felt a niggle of unease. 'Something, I don't know what to this day, made me go downstairs and put Sky News on,' she recalls.

News channels were now confirming an incident at the arena. But early reports blamed everything from malfunctioning pyrotechnics and bursting giant balloons to exploding speakers. Meanwhile, Kelly rang her friend Josh, who had been at the concert. He answered straight away. And his words chilled her to the bone. 'It's a bomb,' he told her.

Separately, my brothers and Gabby set off for Mum's in Bolton – hoping, praying that they'd arrive to find my car outside – and me and Eve inside, apologising for worrying them. 'Where are they? Why isn't Martin answering?' Andy remembers saying crossly.

The TV was on full blast, showing blue, flashing lights lighting up the sky around the arena. As an emergency helpline for relatives flashed up on the screen Gabby dialled the number. 'It was a makeshift helpdesk,' Gabby recalls. 'While I was giving yours and Eve's details the woman on the other end of the phone suddenly started to laugh. "Eee, hang on, love," she'd said, "me pen's just run out. Can you believe that?" Then she'd called across to someone else in the room with her. "*Have you got a pen I can borrow. Mine's just run out… I know!*"' Gabby listened open-mouthed. 'All I kept thinking was, You're wasting my time! I gave the details but honestly thought, We're not going to get anywhere here.'

Gabby and my brothers started ringing around all the hospitals in Manchester. The same anxious words were uttered over and over. 'Yes, that's right. Martin and Eve Hibbert. H. I., double-B, E.R.T.' Between calls, they were desperately flicking between news channels and social media for information. They saw that some families had started to assemble at the Man City Etihad Stadium. 'Should we go there – or stay here?' they fretted.

Suddenly, Mum's phone rang. It was Sarah, Eve's mum. Relief washed over Mum's face. 'They've found Eve,' she said. 'She's at the Children's Hospital.'

My phone had been blasted away from me, but Eve still had her handbag, containing her phone. A policeman had managed to get Sarah's number. 'I'm heading there now,' she told them. 'But speak to him about Martin and he'll try to find him too.'

Gabby spoke quickly. 'Tall, dark, approximately six foot. Oh, and distinctive tattoos all over his arms,' she said. The tattoos definitely helped. Over the years, I've had my fair share of inkings, including Eve's name in Arabic up my left arm, Gabby's initials on my right arm and the Mexican Virgin Mary.

The next half hour, waiting for the police officer to ring back, felt like an eternity. When Gabby slipped upstairs to the loo, Andy turned to Mum and asked. 'Do you think he's dead?' Mum clasped her hands to her mouth and closed her eyes. 'Oh God. Don't say that,' she whimpered. But they all thought it. When Mum's phone finally rang, they all jumped. It was the policeman. A person matching my description had been admitted to Salford Royal Infirmary.

Andy grabbed his keys and the four of them leaped into his car. 'I went through that many red lights I lost count. Quietly, so Mum and Gabby wouldn't hear, I asked Danny the same question, "Do you think he's dead?" Danny didn't answer. He just stared straight ahead biting his fingernails.'

The hospital forecourt was deserted but for a small group of nurses waiting at the entrance to A&E. As if they were expecting families to start arriving. Anxiety gnawed away at Gabby's insides as she hurried towards them and gave my name. One person immediately nodded. 'Follow me, he's upstairs.'

'The relief at hearing those words was incredible,' she recalls. 'We just thought, Phew, we've found him.' Silently, they followed the nurse as she led them through a rabbit warren of starkly lit corridors into a private room. Moments later they were joined by two hospital officials. One explained that I was currently in the resuscitation department. I'd sustained multiple injuries in the blast, had received countless blood transfusions and was very poorly. He hesitated before continuing. One of the injuries had severed my spinal cord. I was paralysed.

'Your mum didn't take the news well,' Gabby recalls. 'She told them, "I don't want to hear that." When they said it again, she said, "I told you – I don't want you saying that."'

Andy interrupted. 'Mum, we have to listen to what they're telling us. We can't just bury our heads.'

Gabby intervened. 'Please, we just want to see him,' she begged. Only two people were allowed in: Gabby and Mum. 'You were lying flat in a hospital bed. Your skin looked yellow, there were wires coming out of you at all angles. And there was a sheet covering you right up to your neck to shield us from your wounds. You were speaking in a whisper. Your first word was "Eve." You kept asking how she was, where she was, was she OK? I told you she was alive. She was at the Children's Hospital and Sarah was with her.' A surgeon came in, Gabby recalls. Mr Saxena. 'He was showing me images on a screen. I could see his mouth moving but nothing was going in.'

We now know that he was explaining the risk of stroke and the need to monitor me before they could operate. In the meantime, there were consent forms that needed to be completed and signed. A nurse took Gabby through all the basics, until, '...and what religion is your husband?' she asked, pen poised. The question stumped Gabby. No one had ever asked her that before. She knew I wasn't particularly religious but how should she word it? 'It was bizarre. For a moment, I completely forgot you were almost dying in a hospital bed. My immediate thought was, I'll ask Martin. He'll know. It was as if someone had asked me what your favourite colour was! As normal as anything, I turned to you in the bed and asked, "Martin – what religion are you?"'

Without even opening my eyes, I whispered two words. *Jedi knight.*'

The memory makes Gabby smile. 'That's when I knew you were going to be OK,' she says now. 'You've always been a massive *Star Wars* fan so I immediately knew it was still "you" in the bed – and there was nothing wrong with your brain!' I can imagine the quizzical looks and murmurs being exchanged amongst the staff. In fact, I'd love to dig out my medical records from that night and see what was actually recorded under religion.

For the next two days, I was allowed two visitors at a time. Gabby and Mum moved into a room at the hospital so they could be with me day and night. When Mum was visiting Eve at Manchester Children's Hospital, others would take her place to support Gabby: my brothers and my friend Karl, who kept Gabby on her toes. When he suggested drawing the Liverpool FC emblem on my arm, she gave an absent smile, until he produced a Sharpie and earnestly began practising on paper. Once she'd vetoed that idea, he'd asked if he could stick the emblem to the ceiling 'so it'll be the first thing he sees when he opens his eyes'.

'I can remember saying, "Karl – he'll have a heart attack on top of everything else!"'

He also wanted to give me a retro hairstyle so I'd think I'd gone back in time when I was finally able to look in the mirror. I'd have done exactly the same if the roles were reversed. In fact, I'd have gone further. I'd have wrestled a United top over him.

Karl was an absolute rock. Gabby and I had spent the weekend prior to the concert with him and his family up in Teesside. He was one of the first people Gabby rang from the hospital. He says, 'I'd heard about the bomb and left a couple of messages asking her to let me know if you and Eve were OK. She rang me back literally screaming down the phone saying, "He's going to die! Eve's going to die!" Karl asked her, 'What do you need and what can I do?' He cancelled everything and sped down.

Tears run down her face now as she recalls how, unable to hold it in any longer, she shared her biggest worry. When doctors first broke the news about my diagnosis, Gabby had just been relieved that I'd survived. But, sitting by my bedside, watching me drifting in and out of consciousness – connected to countless machines – a memory flashed into her mind, triggering an icy wave of dread. Just a few weeks prior to the concert, we'd been cuddled up watching a film together; *Me Before You*, which tells the story of a quadriplegic – a man paralysed from the neck down who has lost the use of all four limbs.

'God, if that ever happened to me, I wouldn't want to live,' I'd declared. It was the same with Christopher Reeve, the *Superman* actor who had ended up paralysed from the neck down after a horse-riding accident. He had been my hero for so many years – it broke my heart to see him, rigid, in a wheelchair after his accident in May 1995. 'Seriously, Gabby, if I'm ever in a situation like that and doctors ask, "Do we keep him alive like this or turn the machine off?" you turn it off. I'll never forgive you if I end up like that.' Then to emphasise my point, I added, 'If I can't feed myself or wipe my own arse, I don't want to be here.'

Remembering those instructions, Gabby was eaten up by worry. 'You hadn't shared those thoughts with anyone else – just me,' she reminds me. 'I didn't want to put that worry on to anyone else. I couldn't tell your mum or your brothers.' Overwhelmed by emotion, she broke down to Karl and told him everything. 'I don't know what to do. What Martin would want me to do,' she sobbed. 'How am I going to tell him he's paralysed?'

Karl listened, then put his arms around her. 'Gabby, let's not worry about this now. We'll deal with it – together. All of us. When the time is right. For now, put it out of your head and focus on Martin.' It was just what Gabby needed to hear and she wiped her eyes gratefully. I'll always be indebted to him for being there.

Doctors gave Gabby the same assurance. 'They kept telling me not to worry – they'd tell you when the time was right. Until then, they advised me to just say, "Everything's fine," if you asked or, "Don't mention it at all," which was easier said than done! But you didn't ask. Ever.'

No, I didn't. Because, deep down, I already had an inkling something wasn't right.

As I lay in intensive care on that first day, surrounded by beeping machines, drifting in and out of consciousness, paramedic Paul Harvey had finished his night shift but was struggling to sleep. After visiting Salford Royal that morning to check how I was he'd found out more about me. Like him, I was in my thirties, a passionate United fan and a proud dad of one daughter. Eve, who I'd been asking about over and over in the ambulance, was currently fighting for her life in Manchester Children's Hospital. He was shocked to discover the extent of my injuries. 'Normally, there are signs and symptoms of spinal cord injury,' he says now. 'But we were so focused on keeping you alive, we had no idea. I remember thinking, Flipping heck – as if he hasn't been through enough, he's severed his spinal cord.'

Paul's seventeen-year-old daughter, Scarlett – named after the Mighty Reds – tells me: 'I let myself in from school and saw Dad at the bottom of the garden just staring into the sky, with his shoulders shaking. I texted Mum at work and said, "I don't know what to do. Dad's at the bottom of the garden... crying."' While Louise headed home, Scarlett tiptoed down the garden. 'Dad?' she said quietly. 'What's up?'

'He didn't say a word,' she recalls. 'He didn't have to. He turned around and put his arms out to me. We hugged for ages.'

7

You'll Never Walk Again

On Thursday 25 May, three days after the bombing, Mr Saxena told my family I was stable enough to undergo surgery. Although I was still gravely ill, he would operate that afternoon to remove the twenty-two separate pieces of shrapnel from my body, starting with the one still embedded in my spinal cord.

As foreign bodies they had to be removed – not only to reduce the risk of infection and allow the wounds to start healing, but so that I could have Magnetic Resonance Imaging (MRI) scans in the future. 'Metalwork in the body rules out MRI scans,' he explains. 'If there's a deterioration in your condition in the future, we can't scan you; we won't know what's happening.'

I was wheeled down that afternoon for the operation which ran into the early hours. Gabby remembers waiting anxiously for news with my mum, brothers and Karl. 'That night seemed to go on for ever,' she says. 'You were still so poorly and weak. We just wanted to hear you were OK.'

Finally, Mr Saxena went to see them. The surgery had gone well. All shrapnel had been removed and I was back in intensive care. But I was at risk of a major stroke. Until the ruptured artery in my neck healed, I would be fed by tube. From now on, it was a case of doctors continuing to watch, scan, monitor and wait.

'It was a tricky operation,' says Mr Saxena. 'As a neurosurgeon, I've been trained to preserve the spinal cord so to see it in that state was not a nice experience. It was very badly damaged – one of the worst cases I've ever dealt with. Both because of the compression to the spine and because of the heat generated when the missile hit. Not only had it hit your T10 vertebra [the tenth vertebra in the thoracic, or middle, section of the spine] but the bone had then broken into pieces, massively damaging the spinal cord.'

There had been some conflict over the best surgery options. Some of his colleagues wanted to fuse the spine but Mr Saxena didn't agree. 'You were going to be spending the rest of your life in a wheelchair so I wanted to maintain axial flexibility. You were young and fit – fusing the spine would limit what you could do.' Eventually, the team agreed on Mr Saxena's suggestion. 'I made a small incision to reach and remove the bolt along with quite a few bits of broken bone, then closed the spinal wound. With the help of colleagues and orthopaedics we then took out all of the bits of metalwork in the rest of your body.'

I'd been left with twenty-two deep, open wounds from head to toe, largely over my back. The injuries were akin to those sustained on a battlefield. I gather that specialists from the Queen Elizabeth Hospital Birmingham, who treated wounded soldiers, were flown up to see me.

My only memory of that Friday is briefly opening my eyes to hear Gabby say, 'You're OK, Martin. And Eve's OK.'

Then Dad saying, 'And Martin, United have won the Europa Cup.' Somewhere deep inside a tiny spark of hope sputtered into life, flickered weakly for a moment. Apparently, I nodded briefly before drifting off again.

A stroke – or a lack of blood to the brain which causes cells and tissue to 'die' – can affect far more than speech and movement down one side of the body. It all depends which part and how much of the brain is affected. If it's a part of the brain that controls the life support system – for instance, breathing – it can be fatal.

On an anniversary of the bombing, Mr Saxena and I were jointly interviewed on the news. We'd become friends by that point, meeting regularly for breakfast and chats. Mr Saxena had reassured me, many times, in his calm manner, that there had never been any serious worries about my health. I'd always been in good hands. I was shocked to hear him say, 'Yes, Martin was very poorly. I can remember sitting on his bed, chatting to him and thinking, This patient could die of a massive stroke at any moment.' In the interview, I literally do a double-take at Mr Saxena. *You what?*

As soon as the cameras had stopped rolling, I turned to him, shocked. '"Could have died at any moment"? You've never told me that!'

Mr Saxena just smiled. 'You didn't need to know,' he said matter-of-factly. He was right. It wouldn't have made any difference. I came through, I survived, and that's all that matters. The injury means I'll always be at a higher risk of a stroke. Along with my spinal condition itself, it's something that I have learned to live with.

I still remember nothing of those days, even though I was conscious for longer periods of time. 'You were on that much medication you were away with the fairies,' Andy laughs now. 'One of the things you kept saying was that your feet were on fire.' I wonder now if that was my brain trying to make sense of the spinal injury? My subconscious warning me, even in those early days, that something wasn't right.

Recently, I gave a motivational talk to the Northern Care Alliance, the trust that looks after hospitals, including Salford Royal. Afterwards, one nurse approached me. 'It's good to see you looking so well, Martin,' she said. She'd been on the team looking after me in intensive care. 'I'll never forget your screams for your daughter. They were horrific. You were shouting and screaming, "Where is she? Where's Eve?"'

I had to blink back tears. These angels looked after me with such tenderness and devotion. Not only did they ensure my heart kept beating, my lungs kept taking in air, but they calmed me, assured me that both I and Eve were in good hands, receiving the best of care. And, no doubt, in hospitals up and down the country NHS staff are doing the same for yet more patients. They really are the most incredible human beings. As soon as I was well enough, I made a point of going back to see them. Many have now become lifelong friends.

Amid the backdrop of reassuring beeps from monitors, I was also vaguely aware of loved ones coming and going, the scraping of chairs as more visitors came and went: my brothers, Steve, Gabby's best friend, Bev, and Mum and Dad, who hadn't spoken since their divorce or seen each other since my wedding. A small part of me is disappointed to have missed out on those moments! I'm touched that so many people cared.

Karl and Steve worked like Trojans, taking it in turns to sit with me so Mum and Gabby could catch up on sleep or freshen up. They're complete opposites but such special men I'm blessed to have in my life. Karl says I'd smile briefly when he told me how I'd just missed a cracking party or the nurses dancing at the end of the bed. He explains now that he saw his role as keeping the mood light – both for me and my family. Time passed interminably slowly otherwise. He'd wear his mask of cheerful optimism until he got into his car for the long drive home. Then he'd cry.

Steve, who has a very strong faith, took on a very different role. He recruited not just his own church, but the entire universe in praying fervently for me and Eve. Apparently, on his first visit – two days after the bombing – I had sobbed as I told him that Eve wasn't going to make it. 'Everyone's praying,' Steve had gently assured me. 'Everyone. We're all here for you.' He is convinced to this day that the prayers played a part in our survival. Even my brother, Andy, joined in. 'I remember walking the dogs and just stopping, looking up at the sky and begging a higher power, "Please help Eve and Martin,"' he admitted recently. 'At times like that, you do pray, don't you?'

Unknown to me, Eve was still at death's door. I've learned since that the coroner's office rang her ward each day for an update on her condition – preparing to make the grim announcement that the total list of fatalities had risen to twenty-three. There were a number of occasions when my family were urgently summoned to her bedside to say their goodbyes as she wasn't expected to see morning. I thank God that I wasn't fully conscious as I don't know how I'd have coped. The guilt and pain that consumed me when I was finally compos mentis, and still eats away at me to this day, has been bad enough.

The atrocity at the arena had triggered an outpouring of love, support and compassion for Manchester. St Ann's Square in the city centre had been turned into an oasis of flowers, candles and teddy bears. Messages flooded in for the city and those caught up in the atrocity. There is one video from that time I can bear to watch. I'm lying flat on my back and Gabby is holding her phone directly above me. 'Hi Martin, hi Eve,' says a familiar voice. I imagine the cogs in my brain back then slowly turning. *I know that voice...* 'It's David Beckham here.' *Wait. What?* My right hand, my good hand, floats upwards, reaching out towards the phone. 'I just want you to know we're really thinking about you at this difficult time. I've heard how much you've been fighting and how tough you've been. I've also heard how you're mad Manchester United fans so I send my love. We're fighting with you and for you and I hope to get to meet you soon. Lots of love. Bye bye.'

For a few seconds, there's stunned silence around my bed. Then Gabby exclaims 'Oh my God,' then louder, 'Oh my *God*. That's amazing.' Then she leans down to gently ask me, 'Do you want me to play it again?'

'Yeah,' I reply in a small voice. I had to rewind the video more than once to make out my next words. 'I could cry'.

Apparently, he'd been on holiday in the middle of a desert somewhere when he was approached to offer a message of support. More personal messages came from legendary former manager

Alex Ferguson and former players Gary Neville, Ryan Giggs, and Paul Scholes. I treasure them all.

Meanwhile, Eve – still in a coma, still fighting for life – had her own set of VIP visitors, including Prince William and Ariana Grande herself, who had returned to Manchester two weeks after the attack to perform in the One Love benefit concert. The singer burst into tears at the sight of my fourteen-year-old daughter fighting for life. Her team rang the ward every week for updates and, that Christmas, she sent Eve a Harrods Christmas hamper with a teddy.

Not all of the attention, however, was quite so welcome. Donations of food and chocolate for families and staff was a lovely gesture. But Gabby was alarmed when members of the public walked into the ward to hand over flowers. Now, they meant well. But in the aftermath of a terrorist attack, your fear, your sense of danger, is on high alert. You're suspicious of everyone. 'All I could think was, What's to stop another terrorist coming onto the ward to finish off the survivors – and their loved ones?'

And then there were the journalists. I'm lucky enough to have worked with some wonderful reporters who have become lifelong friends. They do things respectfully and honestly. But, like any profession, standards can vary. While I was in hospital, journalists were approaching my friends through social media to ask about my injuries. One even went to Eve's school, pretending to be a parent waiting for a child. Eventually, the hospital introduced security measures for visitors and callers and appointed a press liaison officer for families. 'I simply stopped answering the phone or responding to messages,' says Gabby.

One reporter even rang pretending to be my police family liaison officer – meaning I had to be moved to a different part of the hospital. It was extra stress and hassle that we, and all the other families, could have done without – and it was addressed in the later inquiry. Don't get me wrong – I know that journalists have a very important job to do and stories to deliver. But there are ways and means of doing so without using underhand methods or causing upset. Oblivious to all this, I was focusing on my long, slow, road to recovery.

Wound care was laborious and time-consuming. Each injury needed to be 'packed' with a special type of dressing to enable it to heal from the inside out. Without packing, doctors explained, the wound could close before it had healed inside, leading to a risk of serious infection or abscess. And so began the long dressing rigmarole. This involved nurses removing old packing materials (which had soaked up fluid and pus) from inside the wounds and replacing them with fresh material. Each wound needed brand new surgical gloves and equipment to prevent bacteria being transferred. It took four hours in all. And no sooner, it seemed, had the last wound been completed, it was time to start again. I seemed to spend all my time lying on one side or the other, clinging to the side of the bed with my good hand, so that the dressings on my legs, buttocks, back, arms and neck could be changed.

My brothers passed the time in noisy reminiscences about our childhood antics; reminding me of the time I was caught on the porch about to pour a bucket of water over trick-or-treaters; Andy using an extendable fishing rod to knock on the front door when we should have been asleep and poor Grandma falling for the fake cat sick we'd bought at a joke shop. Bless her, she'd even got down on her hands and knees with a bowl of soapy water. There were times I was begging them to stop. But as Andy says, 'It's what we've always done in difficult times – try to make each other laugh!'

Meanwhile, Gabby was worrying herself sick that at any point I'd quietly ask, 'Gabby? Why can't I move my legs?' and push for an honest answer. I had picked up that people around me were walking on eggshells. Being overly cheerful. She was concerned about my reaction when the news was finally broken. 'After everything you'd said about not wanting to be here if you were paralysed…

And then there was your depression.'

Finally, after ten days, doctors decided the time was right. A group of them gathered around my bed that morning wearing solemn expressions. Gabby held my right hand. One doctor held up an X-ray showing the bolt clearly embedded in my spinal cord. He mentioned the words 'spinal cord injury' and 'complete severance of the spinal cord at T10', then: 'Martin, I'm afraid you're paralysed from the waist down. You'll never walk again.'

Gabby's grip tightened. No one spoke for a moment. *So, this is it. This is what they've all been too afraid to tell me.* I took a deep breath and exhaled slowly. 'OK, so what happens now?' I said. There was no crumbling. No tears, no pity, no cries of, 'Why me?' A switch went on inside me. This had happened. These were the cards I'd been dealt. How should I play them? My body might have been broken but, inside, I'd never felt stronger. I've often been asked about that moment. How, and why, I reacted the way I did. It's hard to explain but, even as doctors broke the news, I knew that twenty-two innocent people had lost their lives that night. Countless others, like my daughter and I, had suffered horrendous injuries. Life-changing injuries. But we were alive. We were breathing.

Just a few months earlier I'd been trying to end my life. In the weeks leading up to the concert I was grabbing it – with both hands. Life was a privilege… a gift. We had to live it.

People have often asked me how I came to terms with it so quickly and so well. It's hard to explain but that night, 22 May, I saw hell unleashed on Earth. The horrors I saw, heard and smelled will never, ever leave. Lying on that cold, hard floor, my daughter gasping for breath just metres away, I accepted my fate. I was dying. I'd never see Gabby again. Just a few months after coming so close to ending my life I realised, in those moments, I wanted to live it. I wanted to stay with Gabby, Eve, Mum, my brothers, Alfie. In the last few weeks, EDMR had made me realise how precious life was. It was a gift to be treasured and embraced. We only come around once. Depression had made me ill. But now I'd learned to manage it I wanted to stay here. On this Earth. To open my eyes days later and realise Eve and I were still here, still alive, still breathing, with our loved ones all around me. Well, I'll take that. Thank you. Thank you. Thank you.

OK, life would be different, very different, for both of us. But we'd been saved. We'd survived.

The doctors spoke about support, rehabilitation, physiotherapy, a place at a spinal injuries unit when I was well enough to be transferred. I nodded. 'When do we start?' Just hours later, Gary Dawson from the Spinal Injuries Association (SIA) appeared by my bedside in the snazziest, zippiest wheelchair I'd ever seen. He was a community peer support officer who would help me adjust to my new life. He was a northern lad, just a few years younger than me and I felt an instant connection. Aged just nineteen, he'd severed his spinal cord at T6 in a motorbike accident and been left paralysed from the chest down. Lacking crucial support, he'd spiralled into depression, substance abuse and self-harm, before finally getting the help he needed and discovering wheelchair basketball. As a result, he'd become a volunteer and, finally, an employee of the charity. To help people like me following in his wheel-tracks.

Meeting Gary, that day, was just what I needed. He didn't give me any bullshit about how great life was going to be. He just said it as it was: 'I wasn't there to talk about how this injury had happened or what had happened to Eve. My job was to talk about life after injury and answer your questions. I remember it so, so clearly. I'd wheeled myself in and introduced myself and the family had left us to it. You were still heavily drugged up and had so much polytrauma, or additional trauma, in addition to the spinal cord injury. Most people will have simple broken bones to contend with. But it's different when it's shrapnel wounds. The extent of your injuries meant that how you were moved, how you would turn, everything was affected. You were covered in a honeycomb dressing which protects wounds while enabling them to heal and iodine, which gave you a jaundiced look.

'There were tubes everywhere. Muscle atrophy or wastage kicks in after three days of bed rest – so you'd lost weight. And your body had gone into what we call spinal shock – or loss of power from the site of injury downwards. For instance, because your digestive system had shut down, processing food would have been difficult – so you were being nose-fed.

'I do remember you being quite talkative, which was quite surprising. Sometimes the amount of drugs pumped into people can lead to confusion and you see their eyes sort of glaze over. And yours weren't – you were still quite focused. The conversation was a standard: "This has happened and we don't know what the future is going to hold. But there will be rehabilitation and after rehabilitation, there will be life. Life will be different and hard and difficult and frustrating and there will be tears. But there's also going to be living... walking the dog and going on holidays and driving and sports and recreation and all these other things.

'"There will also be learning to do the simple, day-to-day things that we probably took for granted – getting into the car, going to the shops, cooking, cleaning, changing your bed. Changing the duvet on a king-sized bed is not the easiest thing when you're paralysed from the chest down but it can still be done."

'It's on you, you know; the life that you live, it's up to you. There's no reason why you can't live a good life.'

That final line stayed with me. And that's what I needed to hear. He promised me I wasn't on my own and that he'd visit me every week.

Afterwards, with my right hand, I had a quick rummage through the SIA bag he'd left me. There were leaflets, an SIA pen and an early days booklet – an easy-to-read guide to spinal cord injury, explaining everything from bowel and bladder management to the impact on the nervous system. Exhausted, I fell asleep with the booklet on my bed. Drifting off, I thought of all the things Gary told me he was still able to do – wheelchair basketball, skiing, mountain climbing. I remember thinking just one word. Wow.

That visit made such a difference to how I coped with paralysis. Over the last seven years, Gary has become such a good friend, providing information and reassurance. As I was to learn, spinal cord injury means far more than not being able to walk.

Once I'd woken, questions flew around my head. Until that point it hadn't occurred to me that my bladder, bowel or any other function would be permanently affected. While I was in hospital, an in-dwelling catheter continually drained urine into a bag which was regularly changed. And I vaguely remember being asked to lie on my side in bed so that a suppository could be administered and my bowel emptied. But I'd naively presumed this was just while I was in hospital. Surely things would return to normal once I was up and about?

That night I remember, out of the blue, asking a nurse, 'Will I be able to have a poo normally?'

He nodded: 'Yeah, you should be all right.'

'Will I be able to wee and have sex?'

'Yeah, you know, you'll be fine, mate.'

Reassured, I'd settled back down. Right, so it's just not being able to walk. That was it. But then I did the thing doctors always warn you not to do. I reached for my new iPhone and googled 'T10 complete'.

It was the early hours of the morning when Gabby's phone lit up. 'Martin?' she asked anxiously. 'Is everything OK?'

'We can't have sex. Ever again,' I sobbed. 'I'll never get an erection.'

I was forty; we'd been married for just three years. We were besotted with each other. The thought of never again experiencing intimacy with the woman I loved was soul-destroying.

'Martin,' she said gently. 'Stop. It's fine. We're in this together. I love you. OK? Now, try and sleep and I'll see you in the morning.' Nodding and sniffing, I told her I loved her too. So, so much. More than she'd ever know. Just a few hours later, my beautiful wife, my best friend, my rock, my anchor, my everything, appeared at my bedside. 'Martin, we came so close to losing you. But you're alive, you're here and, right now, that is *all* that matters.' I nodded. She was right.

There was a long road ahead. But with Gabby beside me, and Eve at the other end, waiting for me, I could do this.

8

The Long Road to Recovery

For ten days, I'd been lying still, barely able to even move my head. The only time my view changed was when I was turned onto one side, then the other, for my shrapnel wounds to be dressed.

Now was the start of my recovery. I'd been transferred from intensive care to the High Dependency Unit (HDU). Gary had stoked a fire within me. Yes, life would be different. But I was determined to make the most of it. I owed it to Eve and to the twenty-two who had lost their lives as a result of the suicide bomber.

'Even just the initial visit can help,' Gary agrees. 'Most people don't have any immediate family with a severe disability. So, there's a lot of preconceptions around what it means to be disabled. Some people think, Oh God, I'm gonna need carers… be sat in a horrendous supermarket-style wheelchair. Whereas I turn up in a five-grand wheelchair, holding a takeaway coffee, having driven myself there.'

I remember gazing, enviously, at his polystyrene container. I'd have killed for a cuppa. You can keep your coffee. I'm a tea addict – downing mug after mug of strong Yorkshire tea. And right now, I was gasping, fantasising about the taste. Every day I begged the nurses for a cup of tea. 'Let's see how your scans turn out,' they'd say. Until the ruptured artery had healed sufficiently, normal food and drink were out. Each time I was wheeled down for X-rays and scans, on a rock-hard metal bed that I'll never forget – I'd cross the fingers on my good hand. 'Not yet, Martin,' they'd say apologetically, after yet another scan. 'Maybe in a few days.'

At around that time, my famous Hibbert temper got the better of me. For a few days now, the plaster holding my feeding tube to my nose, had been coming away, flapping loose. I was fed up of pressing it back into place. Gabby was in the middle of a story when I saw red.

'Sod this,' I said mutinously. Before Gabby could stop me, I'd torn the plaster off, took the feeding tube in my right fist and began to pull.

'Martin – stop it!' she screamed, horrified. 'What are you doing?'

Now, I genuinely thought it would be a simple case of tugging and voila, out it would come. But each pull just revealed more tube emerging from my nose. Shrieking, Gabby ran into the corridor calling for help while I continued to pull. On and on it came, like a long piece of spaghetti. By the time Gabby returned with a nurse, I was panting triumphantly. 'There you go,' I said, holding out the offending length of plastic.

'Don't worry,' the nurse assured an appalled Gabby. 'We were due to try him on solids very soon.'

Later that day a scan revealed that, finally, the artery was healing well. 'Good news, Martin,' a nurse announced as I was wheeled back to high dependency. 'You can have that cup of tea.' If my left hand had been working, I'd have rubbed my hands together in delighted anticipation. Result.

That day was a turning point in more ways than one. I didn't just have my cuppa. I had it outside. Al fresco. This was all on a video that Gabby recorded. I have no memory of it happening: I'm outside in the memorial garden. Nurses had fitted an abdominal corset around my middle to help support me before wheeling me outside and slowly, slowly, tilting my bed so that I was almost upright. My legs are akimbo. I'm wearing slippers. A warm, steady, drizzle is falling – even though it is early June. No surprise there. There's a plastic cup of tea in my right hand. It's almost empty. I imagine raising it tentatively to my open lips and sucking on the straw. I can almost taste the hot sweet nectar flooding into my mouth, reviving my taste buds. With a few gulps still left in the bottom of the cup, I turn my face to the skies – revelling in the soft dampness settling on my skin.

'I never thought I'd appreciate Manchester rain so much,' I say. My voice sounds different. Higher. It's an effort to speak. The camera pans around. There's Gabby, smiling, with a friend from my Barclays days, Lee Kibble, and two nurses. Until that point, it had felt as though I was existing in a bubble. In that moment, I'd rejoined the outside world. Felt fresh air. Enjoyed the silence.

It gave me a new appreciation for the great outdoors. Even now, I love to gaze at the clouds. Listen to birdsong. Notice bees hovering around flowers. The old Martin took such things for granted. Got cross when the sound of birds chirping woke him up before the alarm. The new me sees and hears them for the wonders they are. I tentatively tried a yogurt later that day. The cool sensation on my tongue was bliss, as Gabby fed me spoonfuls. My body tolerated it. There were no problems. It was all systems go.

Arrangements were also being made for me to have a very special visitor: since the day we'd got him, eighteen months earlier, Alfie and I had been inseparable. But eleven days ago, I'd patted him goodbye, left the house and never come home.

'Poor Alfie was miserable and losing weight at an alarming rate,' says Gabby. 'I was so worried I took him to the vet who diagnosed separation anxiety. Eventually, I spoke to the doctors and asked if I could arrange a visit. They agreed it was a good idea and would give you a much-needed lift too – as you were still so worried over Eve.'

Again, I have no memory of that day. It's bizarre seeing the moment on film. I'm awake, I'm talking but I have no recollection of it happening. Once more, we're out in the memorial garden. I'm propped upright, covered in a blue sheet, hiding the multitude of wires and tubes still connected to my body. You can hear Alfie yelping and squealing long before you see him. There's the sound of scampering claws on concrete then he flies into the frame – his body and tail shaking furiously – and prepares to dive into my lap.

'I was terrified of him pulling your wires out, so kept having to yank him back,' Gabby recalls. I try to pat him but my left hand is still useless as a result of nerve damage. Then Gabby steers him around to my right side. Finally, my hand connects with his soft, warm fur, his wet nose, his licky tongue. Alfie is yelping and yowling continuously. Sniffing my legs. Trying to nose his way under the sheet. Could he tell that something was different? I'm talking to him in that way only dog owners will understand.

'Where's my Alfie? My baba. My boy. Where've you been – hey?'

Suddenly, my brother Danny has scooped him up and held him in front of me and Alfie's face is inches from mine. I gaze into those brown liquid eyes before being smothered in licks. Gently, holding his head, I lean forward and bury my face in his fur. Even now, I could cry watching that video. My boy. I'd missed him so, so much. Alfie's visit gave us both a lift. Back at home, he was a new dog. Assured and contented.

'Look at you,' Gabby says, watching the clip over my shoulder. 'You're completely shell-shocked. Your eyes are dead. There's nothing there.'

'Er, I'd just been blown up!' I remind her. But she's right. I'm drugged up to the eyeballs and would be for a long time.

Occasionally, the painkillers would wear off and, boy, did I know about it. In HDU, I remember occasionally feeling uncomfortable niggles which quickly became tidal waves of gut-wrenching pain. I've never been stabbed or sliced open with a hot knife but that's what it felt like. I'd wince, grunt, cry out, then scream with pain. Gabby would frantically press the emergency buzzer and run for help. The bliss of new painkillers entered my system – quelling the fires of agony – was indescribable.

After 'graduating' from intensive care and high dependency, I was moved to the major trauma ward. This is where my recovery would really start. On my first day, I was introduced to Stuart Wildman, nurse consultant in major trauma. I took to him immediately. Not only was he always smiling and a northern lad but he was the most caring, thoughtful soul who went above and beyond the call of duty to help his patients, as I was to quickly find out. Then there was my wonderful physiotherapist Caroline Abbott – nicknamed Tigger. Her enthusiasm and energy was infectious. She and Stuart made a brilliant double act. I have no doubt that I owe much of my speedy recovery to those two.

Just as with all the other staff in Salford Royal and every hospital throughout Manchester, what happened on 22 May had a huge impact on them all. Stuart told me afterwards that he'd woken at 3 a.m. to a load of missed calls on his silenced phone. The most recent was from a member of his team. *I'm on my way in.*

'I get goosebumps now thinking about that message. I remember sitting up thinking, Something's happened. Wide awake now, I clicked on the Sky News app and thought, Oh my God. I'd never got to work so quickly in my life.' The first light of dawn was filtering through the sky as he made his way along deserted roads. Meanwhile, Caroline sobbed all the way to work, listening to news updates on her car radio.

At Salford Royal, the major incident policy had kicked in. Everyone had their roles. Stuart's was to make room on his trauma ward for casualties arriving from the arena. Although I wouldn't be arriving on his ward for another few weeks, Stuart knew all about me. 'Every morning, we have a major trauma meeting – looking at the casualties in the hospital. I didn't know your name at that point. We just knew you were a patient in intensive care with life-changing injuries, including a spinal cord injury, that you were very, very ill and your daughter was at Manchester Children's Hospital. That's all I knew. I knew you'd come onto my radar at some point.'

That point came on the weekend of 3 June – ten days after the bombing. 'You were still in the very early stages of recovery,' he reminds me now. 'Your injuries were still healing and your body was adapting to the spinal cord injury. Physiologically, everything changes within the body… how your digestive system works, how the blood supply works, and you also lacked the upper body strength you would need to manage.'

The following day, Ariana Grande's One Love benefit concert was taking place. When my brothers told Stuart we usually got together to watch big events, he made sure it happened. A TV magically appeared and my brothers arrived – with beers (for themselves) and sweets! Stuart allowed them to order in kebabs and then arranged for me to be hoisted into a chair with a girdle to help keep me upright, so that I could feel involved. I remember the manoeuvre was incredibly painful but worth it. I felt as if I was rejoining the human race.

It was surreal watching 55,000 people crowd into Old Trafford Cricket Ground, poignantly holding up 'For Our Angels' placards and singing emotionally along to performers from Ariana herself to Take That and Coldplay. Lines from the songs jumped out at me. 'You know, they won't win,' from 'Don't Dream It's Over', sung tearfully by Ariana and Miley Cyrus and 'Lights will guide you home,' sung by Chris Martin.

Tears pricked my eyes as Ariana launched into 'One Last Time'. The last time I'd heard that song, I'd been standing behind Eve, with my arms fondly wrapped around her, as we belted out the words together. It was just two weeks ago but seemed a world away now. Every fibre of my being yearned to see her, to hug her. But it was impossible… surely?

'If I can make something happen, I will,' Stuart says of organising what happened next. 'As a nurse, I'm mindful that when somebody comes into hospital, they can very quickly feel disempowered. Very quickly. They have meals at a certain time, a ward round with doctors at a certain time, and medication given at a certain time. So, I'm very much about empowering the patient and giving them what they want and need. If somebody wants to do something, I think that – before saying, "No" – you should ask, "Is this feasible? Is this achievable? What are the barriers?" I also knew that you needed to do it. And I needed to do it, as well. You're only two or three years older than me. Your daughter is only a couple of years older than my daughter. I could empathise with you as a dad why you needed to do this. Because if it was me, I'd be exactly the same. Every parental instinct will be kicking in at that point. All you'd want to do is get to that bedside.'

By then, I'd also started sessions with Caroline Abbott, my physiotherapist. 'I'll never forget walking into your room on that first day,' she says. 'It was like Willy Wonka's factory. There were sweets everywhere.' Caroline has a tooth as sweet as mine so we formed an instant bond over giant strawberry Haribos. 'We'd spend the first few minutes of every session going through your new deliveries and deciding what you should request next time!'

Physiotherapy started with the most basic of exercises. Because the spinal cord – the bundle of nerves and fibres that sends and receives signals from the brain – had been completely severed, every single message – from needing a wee to wiggling my toe – could no longer be transmitted. As a result, the T10 injury affected motor and sensory bodily functions below the level of my belly button. The impact was huge. For instance, because I'd lost power in my lower abdominal and intercostal muscles (the muscles between the ribs) – the diaphragm's ability to expand the lungs was affected, leaving me prone to respiratory illness.

'We started with basics like sitting up in bed and controlling blood pressure – using an abdominal binder or corset which wraps around the middle like a soft brace – to offer support and stability and long surgical stockings,' Caroline continues. 'After a few days, we'd move on to sitting balance, improving that wibbly-wobblyness.'

I vaguely remember that the exercises were exhausting – and progress was painstakingly slow. Looking back, Caroline says I was a model patient – motivational and inspiring. But I beg to differ, in those early days at least. To say I'm not the most patient person in the world would be the understatement of the century. Until this point in my life, I'd been cocky and capable. Very few things got the better of me. One of them was ice-skating. I can remember going as a teenager with visions of soaring effortlessly across the ice. Instead, I was like Bambi. While my friends whizzed around, I was clinging to the railings, desperately trying to stay upright. Within ten minutes I was off the rink – stomping furiously up to the skate hire counter in my socks. 'Give us me shoes back,' I remember saying, slamming the offending skates on the counter. 'I'm shit at this.'

My physiotherapy was in that league. My left bicep had been completely torn when a bolt had shot through it. When its dressings were being changed, you could literally see through the other side of the muscle. It had caused severe nerve damage down my arm and into my hand. I remember one of the first exercises was getting my index finger to touch my thumb to make a circle shape. It was impossible. No matter how hard I tried, my finger wouldn't move. To my shame, I definitely recall a few occasions when I saw red. Told anyone around me to fuck off. I couldn't do it. Again, it makes you appreciate these wonderful human beings helping us on the road to recovery even more. They're the ones we lash out at when we're angry, scared, in pain, vulnerable. And still they stay, soothe, calm, encourage, motivate. That's dedication for you. And those videos from my heroes – particularly the one from David Beckham – kept me going during the most difficult, challenging days.

The first time I was propped up into a sitting position, I gulped back rising waves of nausea. Gradually, I managed it for a few seconds. Then minutes. I bum-shuffled to the end of the bed and back – my joy slightly marred by realising I'd smeared poo across the sheet. 'Oh God, I'm so sorry.' But in a flash, the sheet had been whipped away and replaced. 'It's fine – happens all the time,' Caroline assured me.

Mishaps and accidents were something I was going to have to get used to. Learn to manage. But, right now, I had bigger things to focus on. Aware of my yearning to see Eve, Stuart and Caroline put their heads together. He tells me now, 'To get you to Eve's bedside, we needed to think about your seating, your pain relief, your wounds, your bladder and bowel. We also needed to think about whether you'd be physically strong enough to make the journey. The transport to get you there and back.' Finally, Stuart came back to me smiling. Yes, it would take a few days of planning to get me to her hospital, but it could be done. I was going to see Eve.

I gazed up at him in disbelief and awe. 'Really?' I whispered. Tears brimmed then spilled over. Never had the words 'thank you' seemed so inadequate. But there was one more thing. I'd seen the images on TV of St Ann's Square, where I'd worked all those years ago as a young teller for Barclays. Now it was filled with tributes to the victims who had lost their lives. I wanted to lay flowers to them. Could we call there on the way back? Stuart didn't even blink. 'Leave it with us,' he said. He laughs now: 'You really threw a curveball! Visiting St Ann's Square would be even tricker. There were a lot of press around – I was really worried about your confidentiality or someone taking a picture. But you needed to do this and if I could make it happen, I would.'

On the day of the visit, Stuart arrived on the ward in normal clothes and joggers and a hoodie for me too. 'We need to look really inconspicuous,' he said. It was the first time I'd worn proper clothes in three weeks. As I was gently eased into Stuart's clothes I caught sight of the wasted muscles in my thin legs. They already looked so different.

The next few hours, the journey by ambulance, are all a bit of a blur. Stuart tells me that, before going into the intensive care unit at the Children's Hospital, we were greeted by a team of doctors. 'They explained that Eve was still in a coma and desperately poorly, with severe head injuries. They also warned you that she would look very different. She had a tracheotomy to help her breathe. Her head was bandaged and very, very swollen.'

Sarah, Eve's mum, was already there sitting at the beside as Stuart wheeled me into the ward where my brave daughter was hooked up to countless machines, tubes and wires keeping her alive. My overriding memory is of starting to cry and not being able to stop. 'You were able to hold her hand, talk to her and just be a dad again,' Stuart tells me now. 'I never set a time for leaving – we stayed as long as you needed to and felt able to.'

Thinking back to that time now, I imagine the thoughts running around my head on a loop. 'Oh Eve. Eve. Eve. I'm sorry. Daddy's sorry.' Because seven years on, they're the thoughts I live with every minute of every day. At times the waves of guilt, sorrow and regret are so overwhelming I can't catch my breath. They hit me, out of the blue, like a ten-ton truck.

Sarah tells me that, at one point, with Eve's hand still in mine, my head slumped forward. I was asleep. I imagine my breathing, in time with my daughter's. After ten minutes, Sarah tiptoed around the bed and gently put her arms around me. I jolted awake, screaming out in terror and pain. She'd fleetingly brushed one of my wounds.

Before leaving my daughter's bedside, there was one final thing I had to do. 'I want to kiss her,' I'd said. 'I want to kiss Eve.'

'It was going to be difficult but it was clear you weren't leaving without giving your daughter a kiss,' Stuart says now. 'God, I'm choking now thinking about it but all the staff helped. Together, we managed to hoist and support you up into a position where you could lean over. You got to kiss your daughter's cheek.'

I wonder, now, if she sensed me there. Felt my lips and hot tears on her cheek. For a few seconds, I hovered, inhaling my daughter's presence. Then, weeping, I was lowered back into the chair and wheeled out. Deep down, I knew that Eve wasn't expected to make it. I'd just said goodbye to my daughter.

On the way back to Salford, the ambulance driver parked as close as he could to St Ann's Square. 'You had a candle and a message you wanted to lay for Eve,' recalls Stuart. 'The chances of us looking inconspicuous were very slim by that point. We stuck out like a sore thumb. You'd emerged from an ambulance, in a special chair, with two escorts and were still on oxygen. It would have been pretty easy to put two and two together.'

Stuart had tenderly pushed me, clutching my candle and laboriously written note to Eve through the crowd, to the centre of the square. Then he'd lit the candle from another flame and placed my flickering flame and card among the other tributes. I only vaguely remember the overwhelming sight of all these blooms, the sweet fragrance that filled the air, the flickering, dancing flames, the hundreds of shiny, heart-shaped, pink and red balloons bobbing gently in the summer breeze, the 'I heart MCR' signs. The sombre, sorrowful, tearful expressions on the faces of visitors. I thought of Eve, the twenty-two victims, their grieving families. Stuart looked anxiously around for any glances or stares in my direction. But no one batted an eyelid. I imagine him, now, leaning down, asking 'Ready, Martin?' and gently steering me back to the ambulance, to my hospital bed, where I sank into an exhausted, emotional sleep. I will forever be indebted to him for what he did that day.

'It was an honour,' Stuart says now, 'because that day was a turning point in your recovery. Seeing Eve had turned on a switch. Suddenly, you had a new motivation, a goal, a focus, for getting yourself well, into rehab and out of hospital. So you could be there for Eve. Until then, you'd been relatively quiet. Suddenly, you were a different person. It was a case of, "I need to get right for my daughter." You did everything you needed to do. Having those dressings changed must have been painful but you never said, "No." You didn't have a single wound infection – which is testament to the care you got,' he says proudly. In fact, some of the staff nicknamed me 'Wolverine', after the Marvel character with miraculous powers, as my injuries healed so quickly.

I threw myself into physio with a new passion and determination. I had to do this. I had to. We worked on my sitting balance and progressed to sitting on the edge of the bed and transferring from bed to hospital wheelchair using a banana board. This is exactly what it sounds like – a board that looks like a big, yellow banana, that the patient literally slides along. I'm chuffed to hear Caroline say, 'You were an exceptionally motivated patient. Probably the most motivated patient I've ever worked with.'

Awake for longer periods of time, now, I got to know every single person on the ward – both patients and staff. 'Even the housekeeper and cleaner would pop in and chat to you,' Stuart recalls. If I did start to dip, he would find a way to lift my spirits. Give me a shave. Help me shower. Arrange for Gabby to bring Alfie for a visit. Little tiny gestures to make me feel human again.

One video was taken towards the end of my three weeks stay on Stuart's ward. I'm tube-free and dressed in khaki joggers and hoodie. I'm sitting outside in a hospital wheelchair. Meanwhile Gabby is being pulled towards me by a crazed Alfie, straining at the leash. Still yards from my outstretched arms, he takes off, hurls himself through the air and lands in my lap. This time, there's no frantic yanking him back. I scrunch up my face, laughing, as he stands up on his hind legs and smothers me with enthusiastic licks. My boy.

After five weeks at Salford Royal Infirmary, it was time for me to take the next step on my journey. There was a bed for me at the spinal rehabilitation centre in the coastal town of Southport. This would be the final stage of my recovery before rejoining the outside world. I felt choked and apprehensive leaving the sanctuary of Salford. I'd arrived there, broken, at death's door. But I had been tended and cared for by some very special people. I was leaving a different person. Still paralysed and peppered with wounds but resilient and hopeful.

'It's rewarding when you see a patient leave for the next stage of their recovery,' says Stuart now. 'We knew that's where you needed to be. We also knew what your pot of gold was at the end of your rainbow. And that was your daughter. It was nice just to have been a part of that journey for you.'

A few years down the line, when I had the bonkers idea of climbing Kilimanjaro to raise a million pounds for the Spinal Injuries Association, I knew *exactly* who I wanted on my team.

9

Bowels, Bladders and Breakouts

Within three hours of arriving at the North West Regional Spinal Injuries Centre, based at Southport District Hospital, I'd started vomiting.

I remember a flurry of nurses, the waft of cool air from countless electric fans hurriedly plugged in, concerned expressions each time my temperature was taken. A chest X-ray revealed pneumonia. Instead of settling into the rehab ward, I was trundled off to the High Dependency Unit for IV antibiotics and monitoring. Gary and Stuart had been right. A spinal cord injury impacts on so many functions, including the respiratory system.

A few days later, weak and pale, I was returned to the all-male ward. Almost immediately, Gabby visited. 'Am I glad to see you!' I said. I was still under the weather, feeling vulnerable and I missed Salford. Later, before leaving, she stooped to kiss me goodbye. Out of the corner of my eye, I noticed some of the other patients glancing across.

Afterwards a few wheeled across to introduce themselves. 'That your…?' one said, nodding to the door Gabby had just gone through.

'Wife,' I said, beaming proudly.

'Yeah, well you can forget about that now,' he said curtly. My smile faded in a fog of confusion. *I'm sorry?* 'My wife's left me,' he sighed, by way of explanation. '*His* girlfriend's left him,' he said, gesturing to the man on his left, who nodded miserably. 'And his,' he added, gesturing to another in the group, 'hardly visits anymore.' Each face was more dejected than the last. *Bloody hell.*

'Sorry to hear that,' I said, sympathetically. I had nothing to worry about there. Gabby wouldn't leave. But as the day went on, I felt uneasy. *Would she?* That night, I couldn't sleep. Their words had hit home. Why *would* Gabby stay? I was no longer the man she had married just three years ago. The six-foot-tall Martin who had tenderly led her onto the dance floor for our special song was gone for good. Our physical relationship was over. With a whimper, I visualised her taking her wedding ring off. Walking away. My heart twisted and wrenched. Was she visiting me out of duty? Pity?

Next day Gabby could tell something was up. 'I didn't sleep well,' I said. Then I took a deep breath. This was going to kill me but I had to do it. 'All their wives and girlfriends have left them,' I said quickly, gesturing to the rest of the ward. Compassion flooded her face. 'That's so sad.' A few seconds passed. Frustration started to niggle. *Do I have to spell it out?* I took a deep breath. 'So,' I continued, 'if you feel you need to go, I'm giving you a "get out of jail" card,' I said. My voice trailed off. I waited. Would she heave a sigh of relief, pick up her bag and wish me well?

Her hand reached out and took mine. 'Now you listen to me, Martin Hibbert,' she said, firmly, 'we married for better for worse, richer or poorer, *in sickness and in health.* I love you and I'm going nowhere. Do you hear me? We are in this together.'

I gazed down at my lap. Thank God. Thank God. 'Well, if you change your mind,' I continued petulantly, but she shook her head. 'Enough. Now, how was your first night?' The subject was closed.

After Southport Spinal Unit, I'd be going home. Theoretically, at least. Realistically, there was no way we'd be returning to our cottage in Bradford. It was lovely, but completely unsuited to wheelchairs, with narrow doorways, steep stairs and an upstairs bathroom. So, in addition to driving from Bradford to Southport each day, poor Gabby now had to find a new place suitable for a paraplegic husband and dog. There wouldn't be time to sell up first. It meant paying the mortgage while renting. We decided on Bolton, which was closer to Eve.

I threw myself into rehabilitation. I banned family and friends from visiting on weekdays so I could devote myself, one hundred per cent, to my recovery. 'I need to focus. I won't be able to do that if I'm sitting around talking, drinking tea, hugging and crying.' My dressings were still taking hours to change each day, so I was determined not to waste a minute of my sessions. Wheeling myself to the gym for my first session, I expected it to be packed. To my surprise I had the place to myself – with three therapists. Two hours later, sweaty and buzzing with endorphins, I returned to the ward. Some patients were still in bed. Maybe they exercise later on? I thought. But hours passed and the furthest they went was to the bathroom. Next morning, I was up bright and early in my workout gear. 'Anyone coming to the gym?' I called out. Sheets were pulled over heads. Once again, I went on my own. I was baffled.

I know now, through my work with the Spinal Injuries Association, that every patient handles their spinal cord injury (SCI) differently. Some are so shocked by what has happened to them that they become consumed by negativity, to the point that they disengage in therapy. Which, let's face it, is completely understandable. I later got to see my huge file of medical notes and read how doctors were concerned that I hadn't cried or broken down. They were worried I was in denial and heading for a breakdown on the outside. What they didn't realise was that, just a few weeks earlier, lying on that cold, hard, bloody floor, I'd accepted I was dying. To wake up in intensive care and realise I was still alive, still breathing, albeit without working legs, was a bloody miracle. I was alive. *I'll take that, thank you.*

I now accept that my circumstances to others on the ward were also very different. As Gary points out, I sustained my spinal injury in a high-profile terrorist attack. I had top surgeons flying up from Birmingham to assess my injuries. I was pushed to the top of the list for spinal rehabilitation in the same way a soldier returning from battle would have been. Had I been knocked off my bike or paralysed in a car accident, would I have received the same treatment? Coped as well?

Secondly, I had a focus. Eve. She needed me. I had to get well, as quickly as I could, so I could be there for her on *her* journey of recovery. I'd go first, then hold my hand out for her to follow me. When I thought of Eve, it was like wearing blinkers – she was my reason for getting up in the morning, pushing myself to the gym, working myself to the point of exhaustion with my physiotherapists. I didn't want to be wasting away in bed or going over my story. I was also incredibly lucky that the One Love concert raised more than seven million pounds and the We Love Manchester Emergency Fund arranged weekly visits to Eve.

Every Wednesday, the Red Cross would pick me up for the two-hour round journey. I'd sit by her bedside for up to four hours. By now, she was conscious – but still desperately poorly. Her poor head was so, so swollen. Unable to speak or even smile, she'd reach out her hand and clasp mine. Then she'd tap on the back of my hand with her fingers. Tap, tap, tap. Tap, tap, tap. Thinking back to those visits still upsets me. I remember feeling helpless. As a parent, you want to fix anything that is upsetting your child. But there was nothing, *nothing* I could do. Maybe doctors objected to my time away from the ward or the risk of something happening on the journey. On more than one occasion, I was stunned to be told 'get Eve out of your head. You need to focus on yourself. Be number one.' The first time it happened, I stood my ground. 'That is not going to happen. Eve will always be my number one. If Eve doesn't survive, I won't be here.' When it happened a second time, I wasn't so restrained. A red mist rose. 'Oh, fuck off,' I snapped, furiously. The nurse fled – and refused to care for me from then on.

I apologised for my language – but not for the sentiment behind it. No one ever told me to forget about Eve again.

As my upper body strength grew, the physiotherapy tasks grew more challenging. Transferring from my bed into a specialist, tiny, wheelchair – as opposed to the big cumbersome ones we'd used in hospital – was terrifying. I had to completely relearn my centre of gravity to prevent the chair tipping over. Then there was learning to turn the wheels. The number of times I toppled out or trapped a finger in the spoke was ridiculous. I crashed into countless walls, scraped knuckles on misjudged doorways. It was so hard on my hands and wrists, I developed carpal tunnel syndrome and had to wear night splints to ease the pain. But with constant practice, I mastered more advanced skills, learning how to propel myself forwards and backwards, steer left and right, turn around and navigate ramps.

As well as physiotherapy, we were learning to adapt to life with an SCI – with lessons on everything from dressing and washing to navigating our way around a kitchen and supermarket. One task involved buying ingredients and cooking a meal for a member of staff. One of the therapists accompanied me on a shopping trip to Tesco. With a basket on my lap, I chose all the ingredients for chicken pesto pasta (some had to be passed down to me from the shelf, as I couldn't reach) and popped them proudly into the SIA bag Gary had given me all those weeks ago at Salford. Back in the clinic's modified kitchen, where all the appliances were at a wheelchair-friendly height, I hummed contentedly as I got to work – chopping, stirring and serving. 'Voila,' I said, proudly, producing the dish with a flourish. My confidence was growing all the time.

Mastering bladder and bowel management was a completely different matter, however. Until now, I'd been living with an in-dwelling catheter. It meant my urine was continually draining into a bag which was changed regularly. I knew that, at some point, I'd have to manage my bladder myself. That time had now come.

'So, you can continue with the in-dwelling catheter and change the bag yourself...' the therapist began.

I shook my head firmly. 'I am *not* going around with a bag of piss on my leg,' I said stubbornly.

'It's a drainage bag, Martin.'

I interrupted. 'Nope. It's a bag of piss. And I'm not having it.'

'OK,' he conceded. 'So, the other option is for regular, intermittent catheterisation.' This meant regularly inserting a catheter into my bladder to release the urine.

'OK, and how does that work?' I asked. Gabby can still remember the look on my face as the therapist produced a very long, thin, tube and began to explain. My eyes widened. 'You put it *where*?' Yes, with freshly scrubbed hands, I had to insert this long tube into my penis, and then gently push it up the urethra until it reached the bladder. I couldn't feel a thing – but that didn't stop me grimacing and shuddering. Gabby was pretending to look at her phone but her eyes were on stalks. 'I remember thinking, How much further can that go?' she recalls.

'You'll know when it's reached the bladder when you feel resistance,' the nurse said. She was right. There came a point when the tube wouldn't go any further. And, suddenly, liquid was running down the tube into a bag. I'd done it. I was having my first wee in weeks. Once the flow had stopped, I had to gently withdraw the catheter (more wincing), empty the bag of wee into the toilet, then wrap everything up and throw it away. And that was it. 'Well done, Martin. That's your first catheter done.' I felt strangely proud of myself.

Bladder management has been a huge learning curve with lots of mishaps and accidents. Most people without an SCI don't give their bladder a second thought. It alerts you when it's full. When it's empty. When you need to go more often. Or more urgently. But if you have an SCI you don't get any such signals or signs. The bladder releases the sensory messages, they travel so far up the spinal cord then hit a roadblock. My injury. Because they never reach the brain, the body can't respond. I sometimes visualise all these messages congregating around my T10 injury, beeping their horns and shaking their fists at each other. I only know my bladder needs emptying when it's too late. It's up to the patient to pre-empt the emptying.

In the early days, I was like a toddler trying to master potty training. Engrossed in a task, I'd suddenly find myself sitting in a puddle of urine. It was like being a five-year-old in assembly all over again. The embarrassment and shame – at having to head to the bathroom with a nurse to peel off my clothes and help me shower – was all too acute. I learned to set an alarm – and read the subtle warning signs. My legs might twitch. Or my bladder would experience a mini-spasm, leaking a small amount, before giving way to a torrent. Nowadays, I've perfected an almost foolproof system. Every three hours my phone beeps. Wee time. There are also side effects and risks of infection from inserting a foreign object into the body.

But learning to wee was nothing compared to bowels. Until now, my number twos were done for me. I'd curl up on my side, on a disposable sheet, for a laxative suppository to be inserted up my backside. Apparently, my bowels would open like clockwork and the wonderful nurses would clean me up. Job done. If the bowel didn't empty that way, they'd perform 'manual evacuation'. They'd literally use fingers to, ahem, 'go up and get it'. Occasionally, they'd have to push on my stomach, leaving me retching in discomfort. However, rehab meant learning how to empty my bowel myself.

Now, you can always skip this bit. But I feel it's important to explain exactly what spinal cord injury patients have to cope with on a day-to-day basis.

My brother, Andy, was visiting while I was working on this chapter and overheard me explaining my bodily rigmaroles. He looked up aghast. 'What? You can't do a wee like normal?'

I shook my head. 'Er, no,' I replied, bemused.

'What about a poo?' he persisted. The look on his face was priceless. 'I had no idea,' he said, shaking his head. Most people don't. Which is why I wanted to include every detail in this book.

The Peristeen – or transanal irrigation system, which sounds like an intricate watering system for plants – is a tube inserted up the bum and held in place by an inflating balloon so that water can be squirted into the bowel. The water temperature needs to be just right. Too cold can cause stomach cramps; too hot can damage the bowel lining. Once the balloon is deflated and the catheter removed, gravity does the rest, allowing both water and faeces to empty straight into the toilet. Sounds straightforward, doesn't it? However, the bowel needs to be 'trained' in any new system of emptying.

If all goes smoothly, on average it should take around thirty minutes for the bowel to empty completely. However, as I was to find, sometimes nothing happened. Sometimes I came off the toilet before the bowel had finished emptying. Sometimes, I'd be sitting there for hours.

Next time you go for a wee or a poo – enjoy it. Never, ever take it for granted. I can only dream of the days I completed my ablutions in seconds or minutes, leaving me free to get on with the rest of my day. Of all the aspects of spinal cord injury, it's this which has caused me most distress. I've shed more tears than you'd believe possible over toilet mishaps. It still upsets me to this day. I don't think I will ever truly come to terms with it.

The mental aspect of adapting to life with an SCI is just as challenging as the physical side. As Gary says now, 'You experience almost a societal pressure to be the best, to be a Paralympian, to be an athlete, to get back to whatever your life was before. Every day there will be a new goal or challenge. From the very acute days when it could be "Can you pick that cup up?" to the day you feed yourself. Then night-time rolls around, and all your family and friends have gone home. And that's when you start thinking about everything else. How can I walk down the beach holding my partner's hand? How can I have sex? How can I get into a taxi, go out clubbing, go on holiday, go back to work? What are people going to think of me? How will I be a wheelchair user? I'm terrified! These are all the insecurities that weigh so much heavier on your mind than not being able to walk.'

Just when I thought I'd got my head around everything, something else would rear its head. Caroline had already explained that the lack of feeling below my belly button meant good skincare was critical. If anyone without an SCI sits down with their keys or mobile phone in the back pocket or their legs brush against a boiling hot radiator, they quickly know about it. Someone with a spinal cord injury wouldn't feel a thing. Sharp edges or hot surfaces bite or burn the skin without them realising. Even just sitting or lying in the same position could cause a pressure sore to build up. A lack of blood flow, oxygen and nutrients reaching an area of the body could, within hours, lead to a sore. Reduced circulation means that injuries take much longer to heal, if at all. Sores could become ulcers.

Not only did I have to prevent any such breakdown, I had to continually monitor my skin for any signs of early problems, scrupulously dry all my crevices and folds after a shower. Make sure I didn't get too hot or cold (I can't feel anything, remember), prevent dry skin or callouses forming, use cushions to protect bony parts while sleeping and change position regularly while sitting or standing to prevent pressure sores from forming. I was stunned to learn that *Superman* actor Christopher Reeve had died, nine years after the riding accident which had left him paralysed, from complications reportedly associated with an infected pressure ulcer. He was just fifty-two.

Trying to remember every single thing I needed to do was overwhelming. 'It will just become a way of life,' the physios assured me. I hoped so.

Slowly but surely, my confidence started to increase. When family and friends visited, I was encouraged to start going further afield. One afternoon, Steve announced he was taking me to Nando's for lunch. Our get-togethers had traditionally been Nando's and a film. It was too soon for a trip to the cinema. But Steve had got the green light for lunch out, bless him. The hospital loaned him a board to help transfer me from my wheelchair to the passenger seat of his car. I then sat back and enjoyed one of the funniest half-hours of my life, watching Steve wrestle my wheelchair into the back of his highly inappropriate BMW coupe car. Talk about a tonic.

He confesses now that he was terrified throughout the whole lunch. 'You still weren't in a great way and I was worried about dropping you or hurting you,' he says. But it was lovely to be out. Back in a restaurant again. Sitting opposite him, tucking into my favourite double-chicken burger with peri-peri chips, spicy rice and corn on the cob. I almost forgot I was disabled.

A week later, Karl suggested a trip to the local pub. As he pushed me through the doors, I was astonished to find twenty of my old banking friends all clapping and cheering my arrival. I'd never been more touched. My birthday was approaching on 11 July but, mulishly, I decided I wasn't marking the occasion. 'Don't get me anything – not even a card,' I insisted. It's hard to explain but it was almost as if, throughout rehab, I'd put myself on a high pedestal. Up there, I was superhuman. Harnessing powers. Regaining strength. A birthday would only remind me I was human. A mere mortal. I was terrified that if I stepped, or even glanced, down I'd lose my place.

Mum, of course, completely ignored me. Walking with a stick, as she was crippled with arthritis, she arrived laden with gifts, including a new United top and an iPad. I didn't have the heart to tell her off. I did treat myself to a late birthday present, however. Immediately after the bombing, thousands of people queued for Manchester Bee tattoos in return for a donation to the We Love Manchester appeal. I wanted one, too. The Manchester Worker Bee has been an emblem of the city for more than 150 years

– symbolising Mancunians' work ethic and sense of community in the city.

My friend, Kevin Paul – a tattoo artist who has inked celebrities like Ed Sheeran, Rihanna and Harry Styles – agreed to do the honours. I became the first hospital in-patient to have a tattoo. I was on that much painkilling medication that I didn't feel a thing – every cloud and all that. Afterwards, he took a photo so I could see his handiwork in all its glory.

'I love it,' I breathed, admiring the large black-and-white bee across the base of my neck, with the number twenty-two etched on its body. That number is so symbolic: the attack happened on 22 May, twenty-two people died and I was left with twenty-two shrapnel wounds. My deepest wound had twenty-two stitches. I was moved to Southport Spinal Unit on 22 June and my departure date was originally set for 22 August. Some people believe numbers actually link us to celestial beings or angels. On one website I read that the angel number twenty-two is often considered a 'guiding light on one's life path'. Other explanations for this master number included turning dreams into reality and having a purpose in life. As I've already said I'm not religious in the slightest. But, as time went on, I began to believe that Eve and I were saved for a reason that night. I remember saying in early media interviews, 'I don't know what that reason is yet – but I'm sure it will become apparent over time.'

My rehab was going swimmingly. I was pushing the boundaries, smashing it, knocking the ball out of the park. One overriding memory is of me being sat on the floor next to the wheelchair. 'Transferring to a wheelchair is one thing. But you need to know how to get back into it if you fall out,' said my therapist. Within minutes, I was sweating and grunting with the effort of trying to haul myself back into the chair. After an hour, I was told, 'Let's leave it for today, Martin. Not many manage it on their first attempt.'

That just made me even more determined. Sweat trickled down my brow and back, soaking my top. The muscles in my arms and shoulders strained and burned with the effort of heaving myself upwards, only to lose my grip and clatter back onto the floor. I'd take a break, sip water, summon my energy, then try again. Finally, triumphantly exhausted, my arse was in the seat.

With a Batec – an electric scooter device which attached to my wheelchair – I zipped around the ward making 'neeoow' engine noises as I turned sharp corners.

I was also offered a coveted place at Revitalise Sandpipers, a nearby resort that offered respite stays. It was the stepping stone from hospital to going home. It was incredible: I got my own room with lovely lake views and an ensuite bathroom. The downside was that each resident was severely disabled. In the dining room we were all expected to sit together. I had nothing against the other patients, but I didn't want to be reminded or defined by my disability. I wanted to be Martin. Just Martin.

I stopped going for meals. I would order Deliveroo and stay in my room watching TV. Or on a whim, I'd head out to Southport in my Batec. Have an ice-cream on the pier, watching the sea. Or do some shopping at Flannels, a local designer shop. One day, a nurse knocked on my door. 'Martin, you're not eating or socialising and you can't keep leaving the site without telling anyone where you're going.'

I explained how miserable I was feeling. Next morning, she urged me to go down to breakfast. The four spinal patients now had their own individual table. 'Thank you,' I said. It was a tiny gesture but meant a great deal.

On 22 August, I'd be starting my new life in the outside world. I was excited and terrified in equal measure. A few days before, my friend, Lee Freeman, came to visit and took me into Southport for a Slush Puppie. 'You OK, Martin? You look a bit pale.'

'Mmm, I think I'm coming down with a cold,' I replied, giving a shiver.

I had paracetamol with my medication that night but never gave it a second thought. At midnight, I woke dripping with sweat. I was on fire. Dragging myself out of bed, I wheeled myself into the bathroom. Maybe a tepid shower would cool me down. Suddenly, specks appeared before my eyes. And the chair started jerking violently. What the heck? It took a few seconds for me to realise that I was shaking and couldn't stop. I reached for the emergency cord. Staff found me having a full-blown seizure. Before I knew it, I was back in High Dependency attached to countless drips.

'You've got sepsis, Martin,' a nurse told me.

I'd never heard of it, but sepsis is a potentially fatal condition caused by the body overreacting to an infection. There is always a high risk of urinary tract infection when using catheters. Even with scrupulous hygiene, bacteria can enter the urethra and multiply. This spinal cord injury really was the gift that kept giving. My stay was extended by a month.

Recuperating gave me plenty of time for thinking... and googling. I'm a stubborn, determined sod and not one for being told what I can and can't do. So, yes, the doctors had told me I'd never walk again. But how sure were they? I remembered reading about Christopher Reeve's paralysis. He'd set up a foundation for research into spinal injuries. There were brilliant scientists out there. We'd put a man on the moon. Surely someone out there was working on a cure for a spinal cord injury? As anyone knows, once you start googling, you can't stop. You end up down a rabbit warren where one site leads to another. Before long, I'd come across a treatment in Australia called NeuroPhysics Therapy, run by Ken Ware. There were no injections or operations. By using special brain exercises, he was able to get neurons to bypass the site of the injury and form new channels. As a result, sensory and motor neurons were able to run down the spinal cord again. A former athlete called John Maclean, paralysed in a cycling accident, was now walking again. My eyes flew across the screen as I read the words, clicked on videos. *Bloody hell! This is amazing...*

'What's that you're looking at, Martin?'

A member of staff had just appeared at my bedside. 'Look at this!' I said excitedly. 'It's a treatment in Australia that gets paralysed people walking again.'

They glanced at the screen briefly then sighed. 'Put it away, Martin. It's a load of rubbish – giving people like you false hope. Just concentrate on getting better.'

My excitement evaporated. I switched off the iPad. Who was I trying to kid?

In September came the news that Manchester Arena was reopening. All profits would go to the Manchester Memorial Fund to pay for a permanent monument to the victims of the atrocity. Survivors and families of victims were all invited. But Gabby's face fell when I told her. 'You want to go back there?' she asked, incredulously.

I nodded. 'I have to,' I insisted, 'otherwise, the terrorists have won.' The friend who owned the VIP box we'd sat in last time said I could use the entire suite. I invited everyone who had been around my bedside. And then my doctors threw a spanner in the works. 'Absolutely not,' one said, shaking his head. 'You're still on very high doses of morphine. You'll need medical assistance on the night. And it could also be very traumatic – it's far too soon to return to the scene of the attack.'

A mutinous thought was forming. 'It's all sorted,' I assured family and friends. 'I'll see you in there.'

My old banking friend Claire agreed to pick me up. 'Wait at the door,' I said. 'No need for you to come inside.' I pootled along the corridors, smiling and greeting patients and staff. As the exit came into sight, I sped up. Claire was waiting with the engine running. 'Can we be quick? I don't want to be late,' I said. Within seconds, we were on our way. As we drew closer, I could feel nerves swirling. I gazed in silence at the scaffolding and tarpaulin that still covered the affected area of the building. It felt surreal being wheeled through the City Room – across the very spot where my daughter and I had lain, dying. I'd missed dinner and that evening's medication round. But adrenalin and defiance were fizzing through my veins.

There, in the box, were all my loved ones, cheering as Claire wheeled me towards them. Gabby hugged me tightly, then looked around puzzled. 'Where's your doctors?' she asked.

I had the good grace to look embarrassed. 'Erm...' I said sheepishly.

'You've done what?' she shrieked, when I confessed.

I knew she'd have put her foot down had she known. 'It's fine, love,' I insisted. 'I'm here now. They won't even notice I'm gone.'

Gabby sighed. She knows full well that when I've made my mind to do something up an entire army won't stop me.

It's bizarre to look back at pictures. I'm beaming and smiling, surrounded by friends and family – even Kevin the tattoo artist. 'Look, you can see your hospital tag on your wrist,' says Gabby now. 'You're gaunt and your eyes are so dilated they're black. In fact, you look a bit manic, like you're on drugs.'

'I was!' I remind her. 'A shitload!'

Being back was surreal but strangely empowering. There were 14,000 people – the same number who had attended the original concert. Andy Burnham, mayor of Greater Manchester, began with an opening speech – reciting the names of the twenty-two lost in the bombing. Each name was clapped. And an almighty, emotional roar greeted his declaration, 'We are Manchester, a city united, nothing will ever change us, nothing will ever divide us.'

Gabby was a nervous wreck. She kept looking anxiously over her shoulder even while the acts performed, including Noel Gallagher's High Flying Birds and Rick Astley. Karl also struggled. 'We all went to support you. But you can't help being aware of what's gone on just a matter of months before. You're also sat there thinking, Shit, if it happens again, how do we get out?'

I batted away such worries. This was a new start for Manchester. A chance to stick two fingers up to the terrorists and tell them, 'You picked on the wrong city.'

I had to wipe my eyes as iconic Manchester poet Tony Walsh took to the stage to dramatically recite his iconic poem 'This Is The Place' – a homage to Manchester, including the poignant lines:

'And there's hard times again in these streets of our city
But we won't take defeat and we don't want your pity
Because this a place where we stand strong together
With a smile on our face, Mancunians Forever'

I was so proud of Manchester – how it was fighting back. It was 1 a.m. when we arrived back at the clinic. Having missed my evening medication, I was now in a lot of discomfort. As Claire helped me back into my wheelchair, I noticed a group of stern-looking doctors and nurses gathering at the entrance.

'Uh-oh,' I said. 'It's show time.'

Wearily wheeling myself towards them, I called out a cheery 'Evening!'

Silence.

'Get inside, Martin,' said one doctor. 'We'll deal with this in the morning.'

A young Scouse male nurse brought my bedtime medication. 'You're going to get a bollocking but just take it on the chin,' he said.

Next morning, the senior medics didn't hold back. 'What were you thinking? You hadn't taken your medication. You're still getting over sepsis. You had no support. You could have experienced severe emotional trauma.'

I looked at the floor. 'Sorry,' I said, quietly. And I meant it. It was a reckless thing to do. Anything could have happened. And I'm sorry for the worry I caused. Their jobs are difficult enough without patients going AWOL. But I don't regret going.

By now, I was counting down the days to being discharged. (And I'm sure the staff must have been too!) Gabby had had a nightmare trying to find a house suitable for my wheelchair but, finally, she'd struck lucky. 'The landlord said we can put a stairlift in. I've had a quote and they're coming to fit it next week.'

I smiled. 'Great, well done, love. Sorry you've had to do all this on your own.' I couldn't wait to be back in Bolton. Closer to Eve.

But next time she visited, there were dark shadows under Gabby's eyes. Something was wrong. 'The landlord's gone quiet,' she confessed. 'He's not returning any messages.' After a week of silence, the estate agent finally got through. The landlord had changed his mind about taking tenants. The deal was off.

I stared at Gabby in horror as she broke the news. 'But I'm being discharged in two days time!' I said. 'They need the bed for another patient.'

We stared at each other. Not only was I paralysed. I was homeless and paralysed.

Shit.

10

A Whole New World

You may well be thinking, How hard can it be to find a place to live when you're paralysed? Take my word for it. It's hard. Especially with the added complication of a dog. So many friends and relatives offered their homes. But I wouldn't even have got through the front door let alone been able to go to the loo.

We needed somewhere with a downstairs bathroom, ideally a wet room, and bedroom, minimal steps and stairs and an access ramp. It was impossible. With another patient lined up for my bed in the spinal unit, I had to pack up even though I had nowhere to go.

And so began three depressing, miserable weeks at a care home in Preston. I had nothing against the place itself. Both the home and staff were lovely. But the other patients had severe health conditions. There were screams all night, every night. Some doors had 'Do not enter' signs. Dejected, and a bit terrified, I wheeled myself into my room and stayed there for three weeks. I knew if I went outside, even for a bit of fresh air, I wouldn't go back in.

'Your mood was so low — I was worried sick that your depression would return,' Gabby recalls. In the early days after the bombing, she had dug out the number of my old therapist. Thankfully, she'd done such a good job first time around I've never needed to call her. But it was reassuring to know I could reach out if I needed to.

After I'd spent a week in the care home, the estate agent called Gabby. A house in Chorley, just outside Bolton, had just become available. It had a downstairs wet room and bathroom. Would Gabby like to…? 'I'm on my way,' she said, grabbing her tape measure. They didn't even get to warn her about the 'no pets' policy. Having figured out the house was the answer to our prayers, Gabby threw ourselves on the landlord's mercy. They very kindly agreed on one small, well-behaved dog, so long as we had the living room carpets cleaned every month. As Gabby recalls, 'I was that desperate, I'd have taken a shed so long as it allowed a wheelchair and dog inside!'

Moving house at the best of times is stressful enough. Let alone with a paraplegic husband. 'It was hard,' Gabby admits. 'I should have got a removal company but I'm not very good at asking for help. Instead, I hired a van and had a week to pack up and load all our stuff from the old house with the help of my uncle, aunt and best friend, Bev. I know now that I could have, should have, called on more people to help or accepted offers. I think we're both still bad at doing that!'

On her first morning, surrounded by boxes and still struggling to find the kettle, she heard a knock at the door. It was Bev, laden down with bags of groceries. 'I know you keep saying you're fine but you do need help, Gabby,' she said gently, handing them over.

Gabby recalls, 'I burst into grateful tears. She was right. I had no food in and no time to buy anything. She instinctively knew what I needed.'

Just because someone insists they're fine, doesn't mean they are. Tiny practical touches, basic groceries, offers to walk the dog, a prepared dinner, are always, always well received. In those early hospital days in Salford, Gabby didn't have access to a car. But another friend, Claire, who lived in France, dropped everything to return home and help out with lifts. It was thanks to her that Alfie was able to come and visit me.

In late September, on a bright autumnal day, I came 'home'. Six years on, I've yet to use the front door, at the end of a narrow, twisty, crazy-paved path. Instead, I wheel myself in through the side door which leads straight into a roomy kitchen. The floors are mostly hardwood, which is so much better for wheels and I can get into every room without losing the skin on my knuckles. My brothers hoisted me over the threshold and, until a ramp was fitted a couple of months later, I rarely left the house. Once a week they took me to visit Eve at Manchester Children's Hospital. I was just content to be home. With my wife. And Alfie.

However, as I now know, these are the most challenging times for SCI patients. As Gary says, it's when you leave the rehab clinic that the work begins. 'Rehab is strange. You go through it and people think you're rehabilitated. You're not. You've just learned the skills to be able to apply that to within your life. The first day of rehab is the day you go home and start living your life. Suddenly you're the only wheelchair user in your world again. Often your house is not accessible. There's carpet, steps and doorways to contend with. You're in a really inappropriate wheelchair, there's no access to transport, nothing in your diary. The first six months is spent sitting around, putting on weight, doing nothing.'

People with a spinal cord injury will tell you it's the little things that get to you. Like trying to manoeuvre your wheelchair along carpet. The wheels sink into and follow the grain and it's a bit like trying to steer a wonky supermarket trolly – impossible to travel in a straight line. In posh hotels with thick piles, I end up crashing into the walls.

I tried to stay busy and positive. But thoughts, fears and anxieties were always there, hovering on the edges of this new existence. Night-times were the hardest. That's when they whirled up, increased in volume. And then there were the flashbacks. Without warning, images from the night, snapshots, would flash into my head. Suddenly, I'd be back, lying in a growing pool of blood in the City Room, helplessly watching my daughter gasp for breath. What if I'd been killed immediately like so many of the other victims? Or knocked unconscious? Who would have alerted first-aiders that Eve was still breathing? Who would have saved her? Would she still be with us? The thought sent waves of cold dread washing over me.

Then there were the random times of the day or night when I'd be engulfed by guilt and regret. Did people blame me for buying her the ticket? Taking her there? Leaving before the encore? Could I have done anything differently? Could we have run quicker to the car? How did that one bolt get through when I'd shielded Eve from all the others? Why didn't I take it? One more wouldn't have made any difference to me. But it would have made the world of difference to Eve.

Round and round these thoughts swirled on an unbearable loop of self-loathing blame, conducted by Bad Martin. Good Martin would challenge him, fight him off, urge me to hurry to my safe, happy place from the days of EMDR therapy. With a herculean effort, I'd get there. Suddenly, I'd be walking (oh, the irony!) along a sandy beach, hand-in-hand with my wife. Gradually, the tears would stop flowing, my breathing would settle. I'd focus on the next task: planning a visit to Eve, checking my wounds and skin, doing my exercises and physio and getting to grips with the toilet situation.

Going back to work was out of the question for now. Thank God for my wonderful friends who had very kindly set up a fundraising page for donations to ease our financial pressure. Just staying on top of my bodily functions was a full-time job in itself.

I seemed to spend hours sitting on the loo with a tube shoved up either my back passage or penis, waiting for something to happen. The wees weren't too bad. Using a catheter connected to a drainage bag meant I could monitor my, ahem, output – namely the amount and colour. Between 30–500ml is a healthy amount for me while the colour needs to be pale straw. If it's too dark I need to drink more water. Cloudy or smelly urine (sorry, if you're eating while reading), can be an early sign that all is not well in the bladder department and a urinary tract infection could well be brewing.

With trial and error, I established a routine where my last wee of the night was about 9 p.m. Then I set an alarm for 6 a.m. for my first piddle of the day. People with SCIs don't have the luxury of lie-ins!

Managing my bowel was a different matter. Every other morning, with a heavy heart, I'd set up my equipment and head into the bathroom. 'I may be some time,' I'd predict. There's no way someone with an SCI can use a conventional plastic toilet seat. It's too hard and unforgiving – particularly if you could be sitting there for a while. Instead, I had to lift the lid and use my own padded shower chair. Once you've completed the irrigation stage (i.e. squirting water into your bowel), things could happen at any point. So, you can't leave the house until it does. I've lost count of the times I've had to cancel plans – pleading a dicky tum or feeling under the weather.

I'd try to be patient. It takes, on average, thirty minutes for the bowel to clear. But sometimes an hour would crawl by. Another. I'd scroll on my mobile phone. Read a book. 'Nothing's happening,' I'd wail to Gabby when she tapped on the door to ask how I was getting on. 'There's definitely something there but it won't come out.' Sometimes, the water would come flooding out minus the poo. Other times, if faeces were compacted, my bowels would simply absorb the water. So, nothing would come out at all. Sometimes I'd be on and off the loo, trying to have a poo for up to four hours.

At other times, my bowels would open without warning. I'd wake in the night, sense something wasn't right, put the light on and be greeted by a scene straight out of a horror movie. A 'poonami', if you will. There was no way I could spend hours lying in my own wet waste. It would eat into the skin. Cause sores. Risk infection. My poor wife must have been sick of the sound of her name being called morning, noon and night but she never once sighed, snapped or rolled her eyes.

'I'm really sorry,' I'd repeat, as she entered the room, bleary-eyed. She'd always assure me it was fine. These things happened. Patiently, lovingly, she'd strip me, get me onto the toilet and into the shower, clean me up, dry me, get me into fresh pyjamas, strip the bed, load the washing machine and make up a fresh bed. Only for, seconds later, the same thing to happen again.

If you're able-bodied and you have a tummy upset or are about to have an explosion of diarrhoea your body will warn you. You'll feel it happening. Someone with an SCI doesn't get that. We can't even run to the toilet! The first I'll know is when a whiff fills my nostrils. When it's too late. It's already happened.

Knowing what foods will go straight through you or bung you up solidly is also a learning curve. I'm no longer able to eat my beloved peanut M&M's. However, I can eat a kebab or curry without any side effects. Any person with an SCI has their own nightmare story of toileting gone wrong. It can happen on a first date, in a work meeting, on the train. This is the stuff no one talks about. Which is why I've decided to be so brutally honest here.

The spinal injury also impacted our relationship. Gabby and I were sleeping in separate rooms, having initially shared the downstairs bedroom. After five months of sleeping on my own, I loved feeling her beside me again. But I couldn't settle for lots of reasons. I was still riddled with healing wounds. The gentlest of brushes from a cotton sheet could have me yelping with pain. I was even more terrified of sleeping awkwardly and developing a pressure sore on my backside or leg. Her leg draped absently over mine, the dog falling asleep on me – everyday occurrences could trigger skin damage and lead to a dreaded pressure sore. So Gabby and Alfie decamped to the bedroom upstairs – I've never seen the upstairs of our house, but I imagine it's nice!

It was still far too soon in my recovery to even think about the physical side of things. While we were at Southport, the Spinal

Injuries Association (SIA) arranged for us to have a visit from a psychosexual therapist, who explained the ways we could still be 'intimate' (our favourite suggestion was that we should sit opposite each other and twiddle each other's earlobes!). As Gabby says, 'She was lovely but it was all too much, too soon. You were still on morphine and having your wounds packed. It didn't even cross my mind. The fact that you were still here, alive, was all that mattered.' I had to agree. At that time, we had far bigger issues to worry about. But over time we did start to give it more thought.

Even if they won't admit it, people are intrigued by sex – and if a person with an SCI can still manage it. I said I'd be honest so, here goes.

An SCI affects people in different ways. It all depends on the injury, the person and their partner. In my case, there is no feeling or response from the belly button down. So, in the same way as I can't go to the loo normally, I don't experience physical arousal so am unable to get an erection or ejaculate. However, with Viagra I can get and maintain an erection. However, just as with going to the loo, there's no spontaneity. Even now, I yearn for those 'spur of the moment' occasions. Of grabbing Gabby from behind with a playful 'way hay' when she's bent over the dishwasher. It takes a bit of planning and is very different to how things used to be but, yes, we are still able to feel close.

My heart goes out to those patients in the spinal unit whose relationships had fallen apart. I wondered if there were cracks before the injury. Was sex, or lack of it, just one of many insurmountable problems they were faced with? Any illness or condition, not just a spinal cord injury, can take its toll on a relationship. All I know is that I'm the luckiest man in the world to have Gabby by my side.

As you can imagine, there was still huge media interest into the bombing – the deadliest terrorist attack in the country since the '7/7 bombings' – the 7 July attacks – in London in 2005. Police were convinced that suicide bomber Salman Abedi, twenty-two, had not acted alone. Just the day after the attack, his younger brother, Hashem, twenty, was arrested in Libya and extradition applications were put in place. I'd agreed to be interviewed for an ITV *Granada Reports* documentary called *Manchester: 100 Days after the Attack*. It was shown on 30 August 2017, while I was still in hospital. It made for harrowing viewing, featuring interviews with bereaved families and struggling survivors.

As I watched it, there was one line which jumped out at me. I pressed pause and rewound to hear it again. 'Within minutes police and paramedics were on their way...' Cogs inside my brain were clicking, whirring. So why were Eve and I left dying on the floor for so long? I remembered everything on the night so clearly. Asking, over and over, 'Where are the ambulances? Where are they?' and hearing others ask the same. I had no idea how long we were there for. But it wasn't just a few minutes.

So far, I still knew very little about what had happened. The security guard who had treated me in the City Room had visited me while I was at Southport. He explained that I'd eventually been carried out on a piece of hoarding to Victoria station where paramedics were waiting. I remember frowning. Surely the paramedics would have come to us? With stretchers? And if not, why not?

In July, Manchester Mayor Andy Burnham had announced an independent review into the preparedness for, and emergency response to, the attack. It would be chaired by Lord Bob Kerslake. At this point there was no suggestion that a full inquiry was necessary – and I was blissfully unaware of how the shortcomings to the attack response would be concealed. I just thought, Maybe this will provide answers. I was happy to be interviewed for the review. I told them my memories from the night, my concerns about treatment delays and about the makeshift stretchers. The report was due out the following spring. All I could do now was wait.

One week after the *100 Days* documentary aired, I received a message via Facebook Messenger. *Hi Martin I hope you don't mind me contacting you…* Over the last few months, I'd received countless similar messages. Some were from journalists wanting interviews. Others from perfect strangers sending best wishes for a speedy recovery. *I eventually plucked up the courage to watch* Manchester 100 Days On. *I believe I'm one of the paramedics who took you from the arena to Salford Royal.*

Bloody hell! I gazed at his name and profile picture. Nope, not even the faintest ringing of bells. I started typing: 'Hi Paul good to hear from you. I don't remember much from the night. Unfortunately, I can't say I recognise you. But would be good to know what happened from the arena to arriving in hospital as I was unidentified for several hours.' I asked if he could fill in the details.

I waited, nervously. I could see 'Paul is typing'. I hesitated. Did I really want to know this? Would I be opening myself up to trauma? Should I be doing this with the support of a counsellor? Suddenly the screen flashed into life. Unable to help myself, I devoured the words as he talked me through what happened on the night. The following morning, he'd returned to the hospital after his shift finished and was relieved to find I was still alive. Then he explained, *'That's the last I knew until my wife watched this programme last week.'* She had been watching with their daughter, Scarlett, when my name flashed up during an interview. 'Martin!' she'd repeated. 'Isn't that the name of the man your dad looked after?'

She continued to watch avidly. Spinal cord injury, concern about teenage daughter, Salford Royal Infirmary. It had to be the same man, surely? When Paul arrived home from work, she'd shown him my Facebook profile. 'Is this the Martin you looked after that night?'

Paul had paled, then nodded. 'That's him,' he'd replied. It took a week before he could summon the courage to watch the programme.

Then all the pieces fitted together. It was hard to watch but I was so glad to see that you survived those horrific injuries.

I had to wipe my eyes before replying. 'Well, thank you for saving my life. I'm due to be finally released from hospital next week and get to go home. I'm so looking forward to putting the events behind me and trying to get back to some normality.'

We continued to message over the next few weeks. I added him to the list of people I needed to thank in person. Thank-you cards had all been sent but they didn't seem enough.

On 3 October, I received a message on Twitter from a freelance journalist called Fiona Duffy. I've since admitted to her that 99 per cent of messages starting 'I'm a journalist' had immediately been deleted. But something about this one made me continue reading. She'd recently written about a triathlete named Steve Cook who had been paralysed in a cycling accident. The accident happened just weeks after he'd completed his first Ironman. Poor sod. But Steve was currently on his second course of treatment at a NeuroPhysics clinic in Queensland, Australia, and making great progress. I paused. A faint bell of recognition started ringing. Where had I heard of NeuroPhysics? *Steve was inspired to visit after reading about Australian para-athlete John Maclean, who is now walking again after being paralysed for twenty-five years.*

The cogs slotted together. Bingo. That was it! It was the centre I'd been reading about on Google while at Southport. *The clinic director Ken Ware would very much like to speak with you. If you'd like to drop me a line I can put you in touch with him.*

I re-read the message, then put the iPad down. Blimey. I reminded myself what the member of staff at the hospital had said about getting my hopes up. But there was no harm in finding out more, surely? Fiona explained that, while researching the article about Steve Cook, she'd arranged to skype with Ken. Their meeting was at 9 a.m. on 23 May 2017, the day the world was waking to the news of the atrocity. *Ken was really disturbed by the news footage and immediately expressed his condolences, hoping none of my family or friends had been caught up in it.*

Ken explained that Steve was the first, and only, UK person to have been treated at the clinic. He was really keen to work with another UK patient both to raise more awareness of his therapy and expand to other countries. Fiona suggested they work together. Three months on, Fiona watched the Granada documentary and sent a link to Ken. *I'd be happy to arrange a Skype chat*, she suggested.

I showed the messages to Gabby. 'It's worth seeing what he's got to say,' she said. 'You've got nothing to lose.'

Two weeks later I found myself sitting in front of my laptop. It was 9.a.m. UK time, 5 p.m. Australia time. Ken had just finished a long day at the clinic. Taking a deep breath, I clicked the Skype link and heard the familiar musical sound of the connection being made. Suddenly three faces flashed onto the screen; Ken Ware – along with patient Steve Cook who was still having treatment – and Fiona.

Here goes.

Ken, looking tanned and the picture of health, started by saying how sorry he was that Eve and I had been caught up in the bombing. Then he asked me to tell him about my injuries and recovery. I told him everything... my miraculous survival and recovery. My yearning to walk again. My cocky insistence that there was nothing I couldn't do if I put my mind to it. Much later, when I'd got to know him better, he confessed that I came across as 'wired' and 'hyper' – a combination of nerves, medication and the recent media attention. He listened intently, nodding occasionally. Then, in a strong Australian accent he explained how NeuroPhysics Therapy uses breakthrough science to 'tap into' the patient's nervous system and 'reboot' or 'recalibrate' the way it works. There were no drugs, no injections or surgery. Just very simple, supervised exercises on standard gym machines.

'With the patient closing their eyes – to switch off the visual cortex – and entering into a relaxed state the two hemispheres of the brain are encouraged to bilaterally communicate with each other,' he explained. When practised methodically, the actions trigger a remarkable 'self-healing' response in the body. Now in his sixties, he'd discovered the treatment completely by accident while training in the gym thirty years ago. Intrigued and impressed, he'd started to put it into practice while doing rehabilitation work in a hospital and saw astounding results. As a result, he had set up his own clinic.

Over twenty-five years he had helped patients with all sorts of health and medical issues from stroke to cerebral palsy. But his most dramatic results had been seen with patients who had suffered a spinal cord injury. 'The central nervous system, which includes the spinal cord, has a tremendous capacity for self-repair,' explained Ken. 'In patients with spinal cord injury, the system "learns" to bypass the lesion and forge new pathways through the body. As the body responds, we actually see neural activity and movement taking place below the level of the spinal lesion or injury.'

Beside him, Steve was nodding enthusiastically.

'Imagine a huge tree falling across a motorway. Eventually, with enough incentive, and the right conditions in place, drivers will eventually find a way around the obstruction. That's exactly how the body works, too, in the right environment.'

I listened intently. It sounded similar to the medical phenomenon Mr Saxena had explained when other blood vessels had kicked in and taken over from the two damaged arteries in my neck.

'It's quite a radical treatment,' he admitted. 'As a result the hardest part has been educating people and showing that it works. But we now have respect from the scientific community and I speak at international conferences. NeuroPhysics Therapy is fast becoming recognised as an advanced form of training and rehabilitation. When patients come to us, they have usually tried everything else and we are their last hope. However, NPT doesn't automatically work for everyone. The patient has to *want* to make changes to their life and be willing to work. I always need a consultation with them first to see if they'd be suitable,' he said.

Then Steve joined in. Aged fifty-five, he'd suffered an incomplete or partial severance of the spinal cord, after being knocked off his bike in 2015. He'd arrived in Australia in a wheelchair for his first visit in autumn 2016. Six weeks later he was walking with sticks. He was now back for a long-term stay. 'I want to walk, unaided, swim and cycle again,' he said determinedly.

'Wow, it sounds amazing,' I said.

Suddenly, our time was up. Ken thanked us all for joining him and said he'd be in touch. Even if nothing came of it, I was honoured to think my story had touched him.

A few hours later, Fiona emailed. Here goes. I clicked on it, bracing myself for an 'apologies for disappointment' message and dashed hopes. Instead, my heart leaped.

'Good news,' Fiona had written. 'Ken thinks you're an ideal candidate for NPT treatment.' With a yelp of excitement I triumphantly thumped the dining room table. A concerned Gabby came scuttling in to find me rubbing my hands together with delight.

'G'day, sport,' I sang in a ridiculous and very poor aussie accent. 'Do you fancy a trip to Austraylia?'

11

A Miracle Down Under

'This is your captain speaking. We will shortly be starting our descent to Brisbane.' I reached across for Gabby's hand and squeezed it excitedly. This was it. Just four months after my virtual meeting with Ken, I was flying halfway across the world to meet him. Opportunities like this didn't happen very often. I was grabbing it with both hands. I'd been following Ken's advice to stay calm and minimise stress in preparation for the therapy but it had been a whirlwind few months.

After nine months in hospital, Eve, now fifteen, had finally left Manchester Children's Hospital and returned home. A long road lay ahead. She was still non-verbal, being fed by tube and would require care 24/7 for life. Walking, talking and eating would need to be learned all over again, but I had no doubt she'd get there. 'You're a Hibbert,' I reminded her. 'And nothing beats a Hibbert.'

I'd also been rushed back to hospital in December with another bout of sepsis. It looked as if this was going to be my achilles heel. I'd spent the first two months of the year recuperating and getting my strength back.

A few weeks before our trip, Fiona had also arranged for Ken's first UK patient, Steve Cook, to visit us. I watched from the window as his car pulled up. The driver door opened; one foot emerged and placed itself confidently on the pavement, followed by the other. Then there was Steve himself, rising to his full height with a crutch under each arm. Slowly, and deliberately, he made his way up the path to my front door. I heard a sharp intake of breath beside me. Gabby was watching transfixed.

'He's walking!' I gasped, 'Gabby, he's walking.'

I immediately warmed to Steve; slim and athletic with twinkling eyes and a smile that could light up a room. I also recognised that same drive and determination to make the best of the cards he'd been dealt. His cheery demeanour was all down to the therapy, he explained with a bashful shrug. Ken had taught him to accept the accident as a chapter in the past. He was now looking forward. He was reluctant to even talk about it, but briefly explained how, while out cycling, he'd been hit from behind by a car travelling at 60 m.p.h. He'd ricocheted off the windscreen and hit a copse at the side of the road, sustaining horrific injuries, including four spinal fractures. He'd known, instantly, that he was paralysed when the feeling went from his legs.

'They didn't even think I'd make it to hospital,' he said. I nodded. That was just what Paul, the paramedic, had said about me. 'No one ever said, "You'll never walk again." But when they start talking about paraplegia and saying things like, "Chances are nothing's going to come back," you realise, They're breaking the news gently here.'

Like me, he'd been transferred to a spinal unit for rehabilitation. 'I'd been trying to stay positive until my consultant said my chances of recovery were between zero and three per cent. Afterwards, my wife Louise wheeled me into the town centre. Sitting outside a coffee shop, we looked at each other then started to cry. After five minutes we hugged and promised there would be no more tears. I was lucky to have survived – and we'd cope – whatever happened. But I still vowed to be in that tiny percentage who do recover. When you are in a position like this, all you can think is, There's got to be a way out.'

Again, like me, Steve had spent hours googling treatments and came across Ken's clinic. He, too, had been astounded to read about Ken's most high-profile patient – John Maclean – who had been left paralysed from the waist down after being hit by a truck while out cycling at the age of twenty-two. Maclean had become a world-famous Paralympian – scooping a silver medal in rowing at the Beijing Paralympic Games and swimming the English Channel. Then, in 2013, while training for the Rio Paralympics, he'd sought treatment from Ken for an unrelated shoulder injury. As a result of the whole-body therapy, John was astounded to regain movement in his legs. Suddenly, John's focus and goal changed. He decided he wanted to walk holding his wife's hand and pick up his young son. After four days, he was taking unaided steps. Over time he not only smashed his new goals, he completed a triathlon.

'I immediately thought, I'm going there,' Steve told me. He'd spent six weeks with Ken in 2016 and his second trip had lasted six months. 'It's completely different to anything I've ever done. Keep an open mind – have no expectations. I'll be thinking of you.'

Fiona had sent me John Maclean's autobiography *How Far Can You Go?* but I couldn't get beyond the first few pages. The man was a machine, a legend. He'd been a serious athlete even before the horrific accident. Steve had been one of the best time trial cyclists in the UK. They were in a completely different league to me. What if it didn't work? I focused on planning for the trip – applying for visas, booking flights, arranging disabled-friendly hotels and how on earth I'd get my wheelchair out there.

We were stunned at the mountain of essentials: plastic sheets, bowel irrigation and catheter kits, medication, painkillers, digital thermometer, cushions, skin creams. But there was no question of extra baggage allowance. The padded shower chair and wipes weighed a ton so we arranged to hire and buy them out there. I watched nervously as my precious wheelchair disappeared into the hold and I was pushed to my seat on a wheeled 'aisle chair'.

Now, preparing to land on 1 March 2018, I gazed down through the clouds and sent an emotional WhatsApp message to Ken and Fiona. 'In just a few minutes, we'll be landing and I'll be embarking on a new chapter of my life. I have tears in my eyes as I type and can't believe I'm even at this point. Whatever happens thank you so much for this opportunity.' I'd heard horror stories of wheelchairs being left behind or retrieved with tyres missing. It was a relief to be greeted with my faithful chair at the exit.

Ken's remote, tranquil clinic, high up in Bonogin, was a million miles from the bustling, high-rise, surfers' paradise of the Gold Coast, Queensland, where we were staying – and where preparations for the Commonwealth Games were in full swing. Here, it was a different world. Ken kindly allowed me a few minutes to transfer from the taxi into my wheelchair before striding towards me, arms outstretched. 'Hey Martin – welcome. Good to meet you,' he said in a strong Australian accent. Enveloped in his strong, genuine, hug, I instantly felt safe.

Ken wasn't particularly tall and his voice was so soft you strained to hear. But as a former Mr Universe he was stronger than the rest of us put together and had enormous presence. I quickly realised that when I was with Ken, all was well in the world. There was no problem that couldn't be overcome. Over a cuppa, he explained more about his therapy. 'It's different to any other treatment, physiotherapy or intervention,' he said. 'When patients come to us, they have usually tried everything else and we are their last hope. There's a heck of a lot of pressure to perform – but we always do.'

He then tried to explain the therapy as simply as possible. 'Firstly, the human central nervous system is the most complex of all living organisms. Every human brain contains a hundred billion neurons or building blocks. Each neuron can choose to communicate with 10 to 20 per cent of other neurons by sending messages via neurotransmitters. We need these neurons of yours, Martin, to be sending messages most conducive to your recovery. Secondly, the brain also consists of two hemispheres; the left side of the brain controls the right side of the body and vice versa. In a nutshell, NeuroPhysics Therapy involves accessing and perturbing, or disturbing, the nervous system and getting the two sides of the brain to work together.

'As neurons learn to fire differently, new patterns of behaviour begin to emerge and evolve. This behaviour then becomes the "new normal" for the body. The next day, we start with a "blank sheet of paper" and the journey begins to the next level. But it's all about treating the person and not the disorder or injury. A lot of people try to copy us but NPT isn't a toy. There has to be structure and guidance to it, the person has to be suitable for treatment and the right conditions need to be in place. You don't open up the system without having stable and structured information to insert first.

'From then on, it's about using exercises, or what we call grids, to establish new reference points for the body to come back to. Then it's about going home, resting and letting the neurons continue cross-talking and chattering to each other.'

I couldn't wait to get started. By now, I'd peeled off my trainers and socks; although I couldn't feel anything below my belly button Ken explained my feet needed to be grounded and open to sensations.

The clinic looked like a normal gym. I recognised various pieces of equipment. But I quickly realised that this therapy was like nothing else I'd ever experienced. First, we embarked on 'proprioception exercises' to improve body awareness and open up communication between the right and left brain hemispheres. Holding my arms out in front, I closed my eyes and slowly, slowly, aimed to bring my forefingers together. Sounds easy, doesn't it? I'd opened my eyes cockily only to find my fingers miles apart, with one higher than the other. *Oh.* With each renewed attempt, the gap reduced. 'Good, good,' Ken murmured encouragingly.

Already, I felt calmer. In a zone. Nothing existed outside of this room. I clung to Ken as I transferred from my wheelchair to the first machine – a seated row. Although I'd mastered enough upper body strength to transfer from wheelchair to sofa, a lack of core strength left me wobbling uncontrollably when sitting up unsupported. I'd done so well in rehab – exceeding all expectations – but moments like that reminded me of my sheer vulnerability; my reliance on other people. The fact that I was disabled. Expertly, Ken used straps to secure me into a fixed position and prevent me from falling off. My panic evaporated.

'Your legs are very rigid and closing in together – it's a natural protective instinct,' observed Ken. Gently he began to open and close them at the knee. They were stiff and unyielding.

Next, he placed my left hand, then right, onto the machine's handles – and asked me to pull them towards me... slowly. I quickly discovered that my idea of slow was a million times quicker than Ken's. 'Millimetre by millimetre, soften the arms, keep the elbows down,' he murmured. His hands moved quickly over me – gently pressing on my shoulders, neck and trapezius muscles, encouraging the tight, knotted, fibres to relax.

Rewatching the videos I can't believe how tense and rigid I am. My shoulders persistently rise to my ears, my elbows flare out at sharp angles and my head and neck jut forwards. If Ken is despairing at the hard work that lies ahead over the next two weeks, he doesn't show it. Bizarrely, we weren't even working with any weights. It was the slow and precise action of the movements that would get my brain waking up and responding.

It sounds easy. It's not. Your instinct is to strain. Use effort. Having to control the movement, with no weights whatsoever, was like nothing I'd ever done before, requiring both concentration and enormous effort. Even if one side of the body might be stronger than the other, which is often the case, both need to work in perfect harmony – moving a fraction of a distance at a time.

I'd closed my eyes to switch off the visual cortex part of the brain and encourage both hemispheres to communicate in a different way. With a gentle placing of his hands here and there, Ken adjusted my posture and position until the right side completely mirrored my right. To anyone watching it all looked so low-key. But I know now that inside my brain, neurons were stirring, waking up, communicating with each other and preparing to fire.

Watching the video is like seeing poetry in motion. After thirty years of fine-tuning the therapy, Ken knows exactly what he is doing. His eyes are constantly watching, assessing and flickering from me to my reflection, taking in my arms, hands, legs, feet. His hands are continually moving, making minute adjustments and tweaks. These movements might have been tiny but I would soon realise they were to play an enormous part in encouraging messages to bypass the injury or lesion in my spine.

'Seamless movements, with a good sense of self,' he murmured. 'Imagine you're standing tall and strong. Feel that flow right through to your feet. Think of a white sheet of paper, Martin. This is the first thing you've done all day. Let your system relax.' His soporific voice washed over me. I felt I was entering a trance-like state; those lovely few moments when you're hovering between being awake and asleep.

The only sound was the gentle tinkling of the clinic's water feature. After a few reps (or repetitions) Ken asked me to move my hands 'nice and steady' from the handles, let them hang by my sides and lean back towards him at a forty-five-degree angle. I'd only met this remarkable man an hour ago but, already, I trusted him implicitly. If he'd told me to drag myself over hot coals, I'd have done it. However, there was an inner fear. I'm stiff, rigid, unable to let go. My tummy, rounded from nine months of inactivity, protruded through my black T-shirt as I lay back against him. 'Relax, just relax,' he said pushing me upright, leaning me back and then steering me slowly in a circular motion – first anticlockwise, then in reverse.

Slowly, I felt the tension evaporate. 'OK, let's transfer that,' he said, gently easing me back into an upright position. Lazily, I followed his instructions to lift one hand then the other back into the handles and repeat the exercise. Already the difference was incredible. My shoulders and elbows were more relaxed. My chin no longer jutted forwards. 'Feel that energy flowing to your feet,' he instructed.

After a few more minutes, Ken removed my hands and asked me to place my palms together – as if getting ready for a game of rock, paper, scissors. 'Feel skin against skin,' he murmured. 'Apply gentle pressure and just feel the palms together. Let that energy travel through the body.'

Next, we moved to a lateral pull-down machine and performed similar exercises – pulling weightless handles down to my shoulders and back up again. Ken continued to make minute adjustments and corrections with his fingertips, thumbs and palms, tweaking and pressing, ensuring both sides of my body mirrored each other perfectly. 'Seamless movements, sit up nice and straight – chin up – think about the distribution of that energy from head to toe.'

All the time, Ken was watching me and my actions like a hawk. In the video you can clearly see the bolt-shaped scars I will always bear from 22 May 2017. There are two on my lower right leg and one on my left, more peppered down my arms and another on my neck.

Next, Ken encouraged me to adopt a running motion with just my arms. 'Feel it right through to your legs,' he advised. I saw my reflection in the mirror, drove my arms and tried to imagine my legs responding – carrying me forwards the way they'd done for forty-odd years.

Next, we were back to the pull-downs – this time with a tiny amount of weight. Once more, I executed the exercises minutely slowly – eyes closed to focus. 'Much, much better,' he murmured, feeling my looser trapezius muscles. 'Picture yourself standing up feeling strong – feel that sense of dominance, of authority. Open up your traps, stand your ground, chin up.'

Finally, Ken moved me to a third piece of equipment for promoting upper body strength – a chest press. I leaned back gratefully on the back rest as I pushed the weightless handles towards him. At one point, Ken placed his palms on my thin, wasted thighs and gently rocked them outwards and inwards. This time, they moved more easily. 'That's good,' Ken said. 'We have a pretty good picture of what's going on. Later on, when your system is resting and your body feels things, just let it go.'

There was one final exercise. After rocking my legs outwards and inwards, Ken placed the soles of my feet into his hips then stepped towards me so my legs bent – splaying out from the knees – and away from me so they straightened again. I was mesmerised by the sight of my thin, lifeless legs bending and straightening, bending and straightening. 'Just focus on what's taking place,' he said. 'See it, then feel it.' He stood still. 'Now, try and push out.' I closed my eyes and pushed against him. Every fibre of my being strained. Nothing happened. But even just being encouraged to try was refreshing. Ken prides himself in not wrapping his patients in cotton wool. They don't need it. Finally, Ken lifted my heels and 'cycled' my legs before placing my feet back on the floor.

'Good first day, mate,' he smiled, straightening up and patting me on the shoulders.

In just two hours, I was sitting more upright and feeling ten times stronger. 'Rest up now until tomorrow,' Ken advised me. 'The fired-up neurons will continue to chatter to each other long after the session has finished.'

Tiredness crept over me on the drive back to the hotel and I could feel my head nodding. I didn't feel I'd done that much but my brain told me otherwise. That night I was lying on the hotel bed – flicking through TV channels. My bare legs were stretched out on the bed. Already my feet were more upright instead of falling, helpless, out to the sides. I decided to tune in to everything Ken had taught me that day. Put it to the test. I stared at my left big toe.

I was going to tell it to move.

I gazed at it. Switched off from everything else.

Move.

Immediately, the muscles in my left leg rippled. The toe responded.

What the…?

I tried it again.

Move.

It happened again.

I called to Gabby. She emerged, still brushing her teeth. My face was flushed with excitement. 'Watch this,' I said. Her confused gaze followed my pointed finger. 'Move!' I commanded. Then her eyes widened. She stopped brushing. Her expression told me everything I needed to know. I hadn't imagined it. And I wasn't dreaming. My right big toe had just flexed.

12

Standing Tall

Next morning, I wheeled myself quickly into the clinic – bursting
with excitement. Ken smiled encouragingly as I told him my
breakthrough. Then, calmly, serenely, he stressed today was a new
day. We were starting again. 'Blank sheet of paper, remember.
Ready to go?'

After the proprioception exercises, he sat me on the leg curl
machine. Instinctively, I reached for the handles. But, instead, Ken
placed my hands at either end of the machine's red support rollers.
These are usually lowered down on top of the thighs to keep them
in place while the legs perform the leg curl movement. But today,
they were going to be used in a completely different way. Ken
asked me to apply pressure, as if trying to push them together. I
focused. And pressed. Ken's instructions washed over me.

Gradually, I realised a sensation was stirring within me.
Without warning, my head rolled forward then jerked backwards,
as if I'd suddenly dozed off. A judder surged through my body and
I let out an involuntary intake then shuddery exhale of breath.

Ken removed my hands from the roller and asked me to let them
drop. 'Go with it,' he urged gently. To my astonishment, my trunk
began to rock and jerk gently. 'That's it – rock and roll,' Ken said.
'Giddy up. Feel the tipping point and go beyond it. Let the tremors
evolve. Don't judge yourself.' By now, my head was bobbing like

a nodding dog on a car dashboard. My arms floated upwards and remained outstretched – helping to keep me balanced. 'Beautiful, beautiful… your body knows what it's doing. Don't try and be in control. You have got to trust it.'

Then he turned to Gabby and Fiona. 'Can you see how he is self-supporting?' he asked quietly. At one point, Ken lifted the back of my T-shirt to show how my spine was visibly moving below the scar. If I toppled too far forwards or back my bottom shifted in the chair to right itself.

The seat clanged and chimed as I rocked and swayed. Throughout, Ken stood closely behind me, arms outstretched over me like an angel's wings. Even though my eyes were closed, I could sense his presence – knew that he'd step in and catch me if I overbalanced.

After a few more moments of this, the movements subsided. I opened my eyes. As a result of the brain-stimulating exercises I'd just experienced my first 'transitional neurological tremor'. Ken offered a bottle of water and I took it greedily. Taking a generous swig, I swilled it around my parched mouth then swallowed, and handed it back. I couldn't wait to get going again.

'Already you've improved your range of movement and ability to self-support,' Ken commented. 'Take notice of every sensation. You need to override all your natural instincts to respond and react to calm it all down.'

I'm not a scientist but, in a nutshell, Ken's carefully controlled exercises trigger a reaction in the brain. As the nervous system responds, a rhythmic tremor passes through the entire body – causing both torso and limbs to rock and jerk. 'This is a powerful tool which really opens up the central nervous system and speeds up communication,' explained Ken, kneeling down in front of me to reassure me.

'It's a bizarre feeling, like sitting on a bucking bronco,' I told Gabby and Fiona afterwards. 'You just have to relax and go with it. It's as if an internal force is trying to come out but it's not scary at all – in fact, it feels really peaceful.'

Taking my hands, Ken encouraged me to bend from the waist and lean forwards towards him, before returning to the back rest. 'Let's find that tipping point,' he repeated. *Here we go again.* Ken gently cupped my wrists in his hands and, once again, I'm rocking, bucking and swaying – shifting from one buttock to another. 'Let it evolve,' Ken instructed and the movements became more intense and rhythmic. 'That's good, mate,' he said, encouragingly. 'It takes a lot of courage to let yourself go.'

Finally, the tremors subsided. Exhausted, I sat back and opened my eyes. Releasing both emotional restraint and excess energy is a vital part of treatment. At one point I felt a wave of feelings rising. All the pain, hurt, guilt and regret from the last ten months was whirling like a maelstrom inside me. *Oh God, I think I'm going to cry.*

'Let it out,' Ken urged me gently. 'You're in the right place.'

It was like a dam bursting. Sobs racked my body. Fat tears coursed down my face and splashed onto my knees. The release, the relief, was incredible. Ken rested his hands on my shoulders, reassuringly, while I continued to cry. It took me a few moments to realise I was still. It had passed. I felt calm. At peace. Instinctively, I reached for Ken, matched his posture by placing my hands gratefully on his shoulders. Our foreheads met. I've no idea how long we stayed like that while my breathing calmed, my heart rate slowed and settled.

Finally, Ken spoke. 'That was a brave, courageous effort,' he said softly, patting my back. 'Good work, buddy. Now let's go and get some pathways open.'

From that point on my progress was phenomenal. Ken placed my legs into position on the leg curl machine – resting my wasted lower calves on the foam roller. An able-bodied person would push the roller down and backwards – strengthening the hamstring muscles. My legs, however, lay motionless. Gently, Ken began to push on the roller with his hands so that my legs dropped and rose. 'Watch your legs do the work and feel the movement, feel the connection,' he urged.

Then he stepped back. It was my turn. I told my legs to move. The roller moved a fraction. I tried again. It moved fractionally more. I settled myself into a rhythm. Effort. Release. Effort. Release. The bar moved a centimetre, an inch, two inches, then was pushed all the way down. My legs were bending and straightening, bending and straightening.

'Once you see "My legs are moving," a lot more feedback starts to reach the brain,' explained Ken.

Next, I lay on my back on a mat, ankles suspended in TRX straps. Like a puppet master, Ken bobbed and shook my legs up and down and from side to side to encourage movement. Inside my body, neurons were firing, flashing, communicating. I wondered where this was going. Releasing my legs, Ken sat me up so that I was leaning back against him, legs stretched out on the floor.

'Reach down and touch your toes,' he said. With a grunt of effort, I could barely reach my knees. But with each effort, my fingers stretched further. Each time, I reverted back to the sitting position, I felt taller, more upright. 'Feel it, feel it,' Ken urged. 'Imagine yourself feeling tall and strong.'

Next time I sat up something felt different. I could feel fresh air on my back. It took a few seconds to register that Ken was no longer propping me up, supporting me. For the first time in ten months, I was sitting unaided. Inside, muscles and tendons were working like Trojans to keep me balanced. 'This is a huge achievement,' Ken said. I followed his instructions to clap my hands, perform a running action with my arms. There wasn't even the hint of a wobble. 'A lot of things have to occur below the lesion for this to happen, Martin.' Ken smiled.

We weren't finished yet. Ken lay me on my back, then, placing the straps in my hands, asked me to pull myself up into a seated position. I was all over the place – wobbly and veering precariously to each side. 'Come on,' I urged myself. I gritted my teeth and tried again and again. Damp patches spread across my T-shirt. With each attempt, I got higher and more upright. I was doing it!

My final exercise was on the lateral pull-down. As I pulled the bar, my body gently rocked to ensure I kept my balance. Ken lifted the back of my damp T-shirt to show an astounded Gabby and Fiona my entire spine moving. 'That snaking can only happen if messages are getting through,' he said. 'The spinal cord – both above and below the lesion – is working in collaboration.'

Feeling brave now, I leaned back with the handle and continued to lean back until I was flat on the bench. 'Aahh,' I sighed, flexing my upper body from side to side. The relief was incredible. Imagine clambering out of a car after a ten-hour car journey – then multiply that feeling by a thousand. After months of being hunched in a chair it felt great. 'I feel free,' I sighed.

Back at the hotel, I had a much-needed shower and sleep. Later, I tried sitting up unaided. Not only could I do it, but I could lift one knee to my chest while staying balanced.

From day three onwards, Ken was joined by his wife, Nickie, a fellow NPT therapist. They made a dynamic team. On the hip abductor machine, they placed my knees against the pads, then Ken guided them into opening and closing, opening and closing. To my astonishment, my knees continued to operate the machine even after he had removed his hands. 'That's it – punch them out,' he said, as I did five in a row.

Then he turned to Gabby. 'That really gets the neuroscientists scratching their heads,' he laughed. 'They can't work that out. Their theory is, "That phone line's cut. No one's going to answer."' Behind him, I continued to drive the pads out and in, out and in.

On the exercise bike, Ken guided my legs through the pedalling action – then encouraged me to try on my own. I couldn't quite manage a full revolution. 'But you're extremely close,' Ken said encouragingly.

Next, came the biggest challenge so far. The one I'd dreamed of achieving. I was sat on a bench holding onto a horizontal bar at chest height. Ken and Nickie were crouched either side of me.

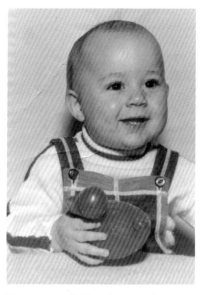

A cute baby – even if I say so myself. Here I am aged approximately eight months.

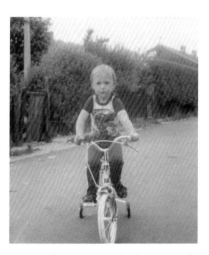

I wore this Superman T-shirt around the clock. Mum would have to wash it overnight so I could wear it again the next morning.

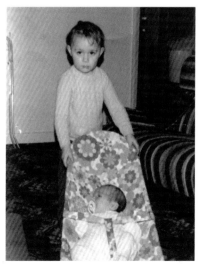

The infamous 'hunger strike' – when I was so jealous of my new baby brother that I refused to eat for ten days.

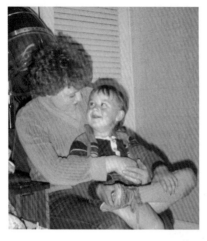

'The look of love'. This is my favourite photo of me and me mum, Janice. I was about four and snuggled on her knee while her 'perm' was setting.

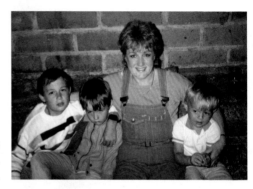

Here's me mum with her boys at a barn dance on holiday in Padstow, Cornwall.

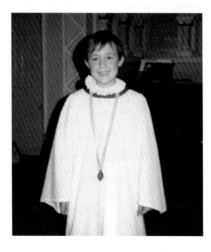

Becoming an official choirboy, with ruffed collar and medal, was one of the proudest days of my life.

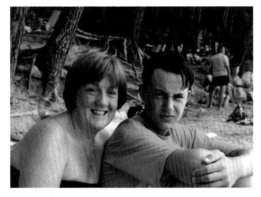

Aged fourteen, with me lovely mum on a rare holiday abroad. I wasn't really a surly teenager – I just hated having to sit still long enough for a photo to be taken.

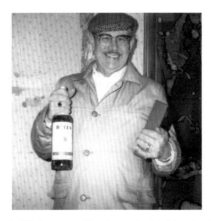

My beloved Grandad Bob – proudly pictured with his winnings from a bowls game. He was my ultimate role model and everything I aspired to be in life.

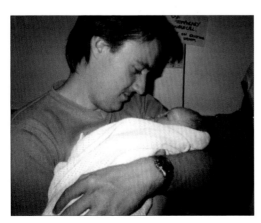

'My girl. My beautiful girl'; cuddling a newborn Eve in October 2002.

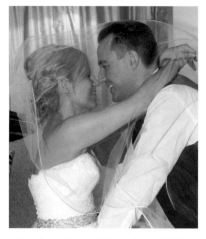

Our favourite wedding photo. Under Gabby's veil, we felt cocooned in our own little bubble of happiness.

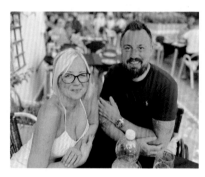

With my soulmate Gabby, on holiday in Murcia.

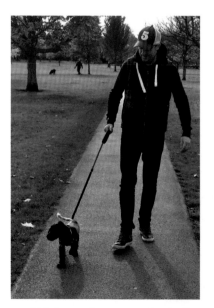

Alfie's first walk at ten weeks. I still miss our long treks.

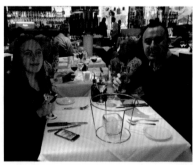

Hours from disaster. Eve and I enjoying our pre-concert meal on 22 May 2017.

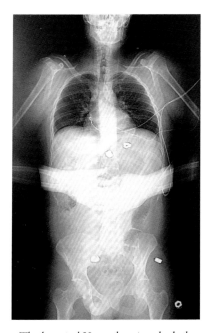

The hospital X-ray showing the bolt that severed my spinal cord. Medics compared my injuries to being shot twenty-two times at point-blank range.

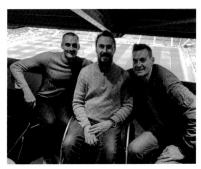

'Play it again.' In intensive care watching a 'get well' video from my Manchester United hero David Beckham. I still play the recording when I need a mood lift.

Returning to Old Trafford – just two days after leaving hospital – with brothers Danny, left, and Andy, right.

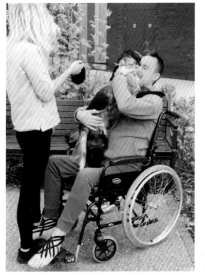

An emotional reunion with Alfie outside Salford Royal Infirmary.

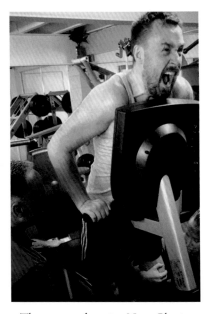

The roar: undergoing NeuroPhysics Therapy in Australia, in March 2018, with therapists Ken and Nickie Ware.

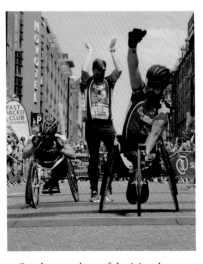

On the start line of the Manchester 10k in May 2018 – twelve months after the bombing. My defiant gesture says it all.

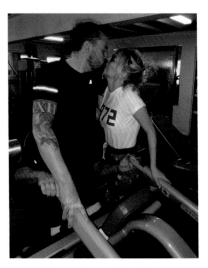

Standing to kiss Gabby, during my second course of NPT in Australia, was a proud moment.

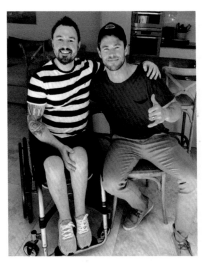

Meeting Hollywood icon, Chris Hemsworth, in Australia, summer 2019.

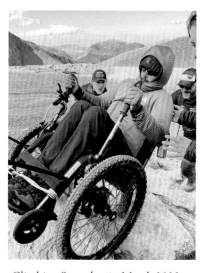

Climbing Snowdon in March 2022 as part of my training for Kilimanjaro.

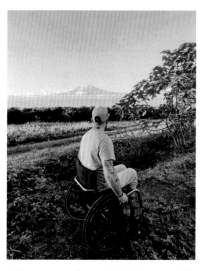

'I'm coming for you.' Nothing would stop me reaching the summit of Mount Kilimanjaro.

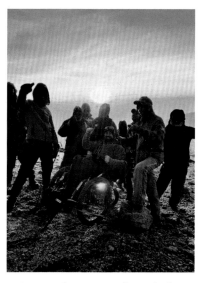

A magical sunrise just hours before reaching the summit. I really did feel on top of the world.

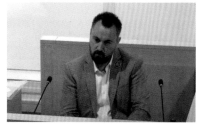

Giving evidence to the Manchester Arena Inquiry.

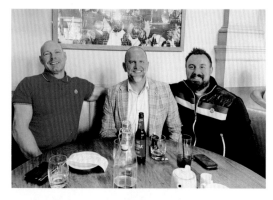

Lifelong friends Steve (left) and Karl have been by my side at every moment.

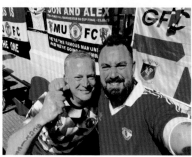

Enjoying the 2023 FA Cup Final with fellow United fan Paul Harvey – the paramedic who saved my life. (Sadly, we didn't win!)

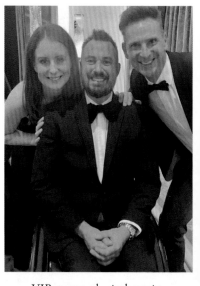

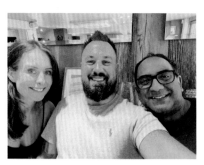

A 'thank you' breakfast with neurosurgeon Mr Ankur Saxena and physiotherapist Caroline Abbott. Thanks to them I'm climbing mountains.

VIP guests: physiotherapist Caroline Abbott and my nurse consultant in major trauma, Stuart Wildman, at a black-tie fundraising event.

'OK, Martin, you're going to try and pull yourself into a standing position,' Ken said.

I look at him. *You're kidding, right?*

'Centre yourself up and push your legs through looking strong and purposeful,' he instructed. 'You just call three and on three you'll be up.'

I closed my eyes and focused on the task in hand. Harnessed my energy. Visualised this happening. *Come on, Martin.* My grip tightened. Here goes. 'One,' I called. 'Two... Three!' And bloody hell – I was up. For a few seconds my legs wobbled like a newborn fawn's before straightening confidently.

'Happy days,' said Ken. His voice sounded miles away below me. I was standing. I was standing.

I followed his instructions to look around at the view. To take in all of the details of the clinic from this new angle. I could see the tops of the machines for the first time. Gabby was looking up at me, open-mouthed. I managed a few more seconds before slowly lowering myself down. 'Wow,' I gasped in disbelief. Had that really just happened?

On my second attempt, I held the position for a few moments longer. 'I've not been up for a long time,' I said, beaming. 'I feel tall.'

Gabby told them how I'd loved being in the standing frame at the spinal injuries unit. 'He'd be in it for hours every day, looking out at the swans, boaters and jet skis on the lake. We've tried to get one since but can't. It's so frustrating.'

By my third attempt, my legs were already looking stronger and steadier.

Next, it was time for a succession of quick-fire moves: 'Jump!' instructed Ken and, like a shot, I was up on my feet. After two sets of five repetitions, Ken patted my sweat-drenched back. 'It doesn't come much sweeter than that,' he said. As the session finished he reminded me, 'We are not miracle workers. We provide all the information and tools but, at the end of the day, you are the only person who can do this.'

Suddenly, it was Thursday – the last session of the week. On the abductor machine – driving my knees out and in – I no longer needed to hold onto the handles by my sides. 'This is a much higher level,' said Ken. 'There is no momentum – all the movement is coming from your legs.' I finished my reps then looked up at Ken for approval. 'Beautiful stuff – bloody awesome, mate,' said Ken. He put out his hand and we high-fived.

Next, it was the leg press machine. My feet were placed against the plate, with my legs bent. 'Now, this is the Olympic Games of leg pressing – the final,' said Ken, encouraging me to push against the plate and drive it away, straightening my legs. 'Come on,' he said. 'You can see it… you can see it.' My legs started to straighten, pushing the plate away from me by a fraction, then another. *Come on. Come on!* With a triumphant roar, my legs straightened fully. 'Really give in to that power from now on,' Ken enthused. 'From little things big things grow.'

Standing was easier now as a result of exercises to release tightness in my hips. For a split second, I even managed to remove one, then both, hands from the bar. After more efforts on the seated row and chest press machines, I was ready to drop.

After all the exertions of the previous four days, I was glad of a day off on the Friday. Over the weekend, Gabby and I headed to a local wildlife park to feed kangaroos and cuddle koalas. I treasure the photos taken from that day. You can see the excitement, the joy in my face. This really was the trip of a lifetime.

Week Two was spent building on the foundations we'd laid in Week One. On the leg press I was pushing a 30 per cent increase in weights. And on a 'timed stand' Ken grinned as he looked at his stopwatch. 'Fifty three seconds,' he declared. Immediately, I felt disappointed that it wasn't a minute!

Physical shifts weren't the only things happening inside my body. I'd just mastered shuffling backwards on my bottom

– driving my arms – and even managed four bunny hops when, from nowhere, I was utterly floored by emotion. Fear, regret, frustration, anger, fury… every single negative feeling was there. It started in my toes and like a Mexican wave, rose – growing stronger and stronger. Suddenly, I crumpled. Crying uncontrollably. Gabby dropped to her knees and gathered me. 'I hate it,' I heard myself saying.

'Hate what?' she asked gently.

I gestured furiously to my legs. 'This!' I was sobbing so much I was hyperventilating. My voice was muffled against her T-shirt. I had to spit the words out. 'I hate being in a wheelchair. I feel useless.'

She rocked me. 'Martin, you're doing amazingly and I'm so proud of you,' she said.

I allowed myself to be held. Ken was watching me closely. The wave that had crashed over me had lost its energy now. Its power. It was sliding away down the beach. It had gone.

For a few moments no one spoke. Then Ken said, 'You've had to suppress a whole heap of stuff. You've had to front up and put on a brave face and learn a whole new set of social skills. Your system doesn't know what the hell is going on but it knows what it's like to be suppressed. Be the real person you are. Deal?'

I give a watery smile. 'Deal,' I replied, wiping my eyes. We shook hands.

Ken had one more task; something he habitually does with patients after an emotional day. 'This is an exercise to show the power of the mind,' he said. He stood a 20-cent coin on its side then took a half-filled glass of water. 'I'm going to balance this glass at a forty-five degree angle on its side against the coin,' he announced.

I raised my eyebrows. Good luck with that, mate.

He focused intently, leaned the glass on its side, against the coin. Then very gently he removed one hand, then the other. The glass balanced perfectly. Bloody hell. He righted the glass then slid it across the table to me. 'Your turn,' he said gently.

I looked at him incredulously. His expression never changed. That Hibbert determination and competitiveness surged within me. If Ken could do it, I could, surely? Biting my lip in concentration, I leaned the glass against the edge of the coin. But any attempt to release it was useless.

'Just think about it and focus,' said Ken gently. 'Clear your mind, get rid of all that noise and those negative beliefs and find that sweet spot.'

Seconds, then minutes passed as I performed attempt after attempt. *I am not giving up. I am not giving up.* Suddenly, something shifted. The glass seemed to be balancing on its own. Holding my breath, I removed one hand, then the other. They hovered, ready to respond. But the glass remained perfectly, beautifully balanced against the coin. We all stared at it. Held onto the moment. Even when I punched the air it stayed in place!

Ken smiled as he stood the glass up. 'That's the focus you need,' he said, handing over the coin as a memento.

As the week progressed, the successes came thick and fast. I was now pushing a 150 per cent increase in weights on the leg abductor machine. Conversely, on the lateral pull-down machine I was working with fewer and fewer weights – making it harder to rise from a lying down to sitting position. Lying on a mat, I found I could cross and uncross my legs – flinging one across the other.

After the sixth day, I slept for a solid seventeen hours. 'That's brilliant – all that repairing in the body can only happen while you're sleeping,' Ken told me the next morning.

When tasks got tough, Ken would urge me to remember the glass of water task. 'This is the driver,' he'd say, tapping his head. 'It's mental as well as physical.'

At one point, we moved to the exercise bike to pick up where we left off in the previous week. But no matter how hard I tried the pedals wouldn't turn a full revolution. I would get halfway. My feet would slip off. Ken could see me getting frustrated. 'I am not going to let this beat me!' I panted.

'Use that anger!' Ken suddenly ordered. 'Come on, Martin. No more Mr Nice Guy.'

It was like poking a bear with a stick. With a roar, I summoned every ounce of energy within my being. Everyone stared astonished as my feet drove one, then two, revolutions of the pedals. I was dripping with sweat but refused to finish just yet. 'Just one more,' I gasped. It was like being back at physiotherapy.

Suddenly, it was day eight. My final day of treatment. I was determined to give it everything today. Pedalling was suddenly so much easier. Ken explained that messages were both descending from, and ascending to, the brain. 'All those messages are flying up and down, crossing over, bumping into each other on the way. You just have to give that information time to settle.'

Lifting my feet off the pedals, and onto the floor, Ken encouraged me to pull myself into a standing position. The position of the handles at navel height was so much more challenging than the bench stand, where I'd held onto a bar. Initially, my backside only lifted a fraction from the seat. 'Feel it, feel it,' urged Ken. Closing my eyes I paused, took deep breaths. Then with an ear-splitting roar I pulled myself to a standing position and continued to yell as I stayed on my feet.

Finally, I was slumped back on the seat – exhausted but triumphant. 'That felt great,' I panted. Fiona captured every moment on video.

More exercises followed. I managed log rolls – from back to front. Then front to back. To the left. Then the right. Then I was helped onto my hands and knees. 'Hold the position,' Ken said. 'Feel that strength from your hips working through your body.' I sighed with blissful relief as I rocked myself forwards and backwards, then twisted my backside from side to side. Then, without any prompting, I instinctively started to crawl. One hand, one knee, the other hand, the other knee. I reached the next mat, then the next. Finally, exhausted and elated, I lowered myself onto my belly.

'A good day at the office,' said a delighted Ken, patting me on the back.

I felt choked leaving the clinic for the final time that day – all of us proudly wearing our NPT T-shirts, gifts from Ken. 'Thank you,' I sniffed, embracing Ken and Nickie for the final time. 'You have worked miracles.'

Back at the spinal unit it had been a triumph just to get in and out of bed. I was in a different world now – but it was the same brain doing it. Ken had given me the platform and the belief to do it.

And this was just the start…

13

Read All About It

It was a very different Martin Hibbert who returned to the UK on a freezing cold March morning. The NPT therapy had done far more than help me sit up taller, feel stronger and realise my potential. It had also helped me process and release a lot of the trauma and pain I'd been bottling up and holding in since 22 May 2017.

As Ken said, I'd put on a brave face. Never truly dealt with the enormity of what had happened on the night – both to me and Eve. Now, I'd not only come to terms with it, but I felt settled. At peace. I wanted to shout about it from the rooftops. And I was going to. The *Daily Mirror* had flown Fiona out to follow my progress in painstaking detail. I couldn't wait for the story to run.

On my first evening back, I shook off my jetlag, showered, put on my best dinner suit, then headed to the Kimpton Clocktower hotel in Manchester city centre. There, in the conference room, I smiled and shook hands, hoping people wouldn't notice my trembling hands. As coffee was served, someone whispered: 'You're on.'

'Ladies and gentlemen,' the host announced. 'It's time to welcome your after-dinner speaker. Please put your hands together for Martin Hibbert.'

As applause rang out, I wheeled myself onto the stage and took a deep breath. 'Good evening, everyone. On 22 May last year, I took my daughter, Eve, to see Ariana Grande at the Manchester Arena...'

Hundreds of delegates attending the Spinal Injuries Association's annual fundraising dinner listened transfixed as I told my story from start to finish. How we'd been just six metres from the suicide bomber when he detonated his device; our life-changing injuries, our battle to stay alive. And our staggering recoveries – with the support from charities like the SIA. Every time I mentioned the charity's name, you could literally feel pride swelling in the room. Many of the people attending were directly involved in the charity. Others were fervent supporters.

'The SIA and Gary in particular were godsends. I could not have done it without you,' I concluded. Afterwards, people came up to thank me, shake my hand, wish me and Eve well.

How on earth had I become a public speaker? It had all begun a few months earlier when I'd made a visit to my old colleagues at Barclays. I hadn't worked there for many years but I'd kept in contact with many old workmates. They, along with so many others, had sent supportive messages. Once I was well enough, I wanted to go back and thank them in person. My former boss asked if I'd say a few words and before I knew it there were fifty people gathered to hear me. I recognised some faces. Others were new employees who'd heard what had happened and wanted to meet me. I had nothing prepared but, miraculously, the words just flowed. Eyes glistened when I told how I'd battled to stay alive for long enough to know Eve had been taken out, how I'd accepted death, told the security guard to tell Gabby I loved her. How I'd woken in intensive care – stunned that I was still alive. How I was grateful to still be here; determined to stick two fingers up to terrorists like Salman Abedi and show that they'd picked on the wrong city; and would grab life by the scruff of the neck and live it to the full – in honour of the twenty-two who didn't survive that night.

'Thank you for listening and thank you for being there,' I concluded. One person started clapping. Others joined in until the applause was deafening. I smiled bashfully.

My old boss at RBS and a friend who worked in recruitment asked if I'd do a similar presentation. Each time, I wheeled myself to the front of bigger rooms, larger audiences. I'd done presentations in the banking world. But it was all numbers and figures. Nothing as personal as this. I found the talks therapeutic. Speaking about that night helped me process it that little bit more. I also like to think that people found my words inspirational: 'but by fighting back and staying strong, we're showing the terrorists that they can't win. They won't win. We're united. We're strong. Stronger than we know.'

Fiona emailed me an advance pdf of her *Mirror* story. I nearly choked on my cuppa. *Bloody hell!* I was the front-page story for the following morning. Under the headline MIRACLE OF BOMB VICTIM, was a huge picture of me standing tall, face contorted with effort, with Ken and Nickie crouched down beside me. PARALYSED DAD'S WALKING HOPE. A strapline read, 'Shredded by shrapnel at Manchester, he gets movement back in his legs.' Their two-page inside spread outlined the therapy I'd had with Ken and my dreams of walking again. The main picture showed me laughing while I pressed my feet into Ken's hips: 'After my toes moved for the first time, every day has brought a new miracle.' At the end was a caption, 'Tomorrow: read Martin's diary of hope.' *Wow.*

Soon my phone started ringing and never stopped. Requests for interviews came thick and fast as the story appeared in all the national newspapers from *The Times* ('Manchester bombing survivor Martin Hibbert defies doctors to regain use of his legs') to the *Sun* ('Bomb victim's hope: dad paralysed in Manchester bombing has movement back in his legs after moving to Australia for groundbreaking treatment'). I appeared on the sofa on *Good Morning Britain* and chatted on Talk Radio. *The One Show* asked if they could do a special programme.

Ken had a hundred emails from people in the UK wanting to find out more about the therapy. Within the first week, the number had soared to three hundred. I was flying the flag for NPT and couldn't have been prouder.

Just two days later, there was more media interest when Lord Kerslake's report into the attack was published. I was keen to see what the findings would be. Over the last few months I'd become increasingly concerned and uncomfortable at what I was reading about the emergency services' response on the night. Survivors and families of victims had been receiving regular updates from Greater Manchester Police (GMP) family liaison officers and, early in January, the force revealed that seventy-four members of the police, rail and security staff were to be honoured at an awards ceremony at Manchester town hall. This was for their 'extraordinary acts of bravery in the immediate aftermath of the Manchester Arena terrorist attack'.

I'd felt my first niggle of discomfort as I read coverage in the local papers and on the Sky News website. They told how staff had raced to the scene to deliver first aid and evacuate casualties. I re-read that part again. Something wasn't right. If they did such a good job why were Eve and I left bleeding to death on the floor for such a long time? Why were there hardly any paramedics in the room with us? Why were we all asking over and over where the ambulances were?

Printing off the Kerslake report now, I hoped it would finally answer my questions. Within minutes of beginning to read, I'd turned back to the cover to check the title. Was he talking about the same event? 'There is a lot to be proud of in the response [to the attack],' Lord Kerslake had written in the executive summary. 'Police and ambulance personnel were very rapidly on the scene and there followed a remarkably fast deployment of armed officers to secure the area and Ambulance staff to attend to the wounded.'

Really? So why were Eve and I were on the floor of the arena for almost an hour?

On the following page he acknowledged that 'the Greater Manchester Fire and Rescue Service did not arrive at the scene and therefore played no meaningful role in the response to the attack for nearly two hours'. At one point, he even suggested that the gap in getting casualties to hospitals helped medics prepare for their arrival. Gabby found me sitting in stunned silence. 'This is bullshit,' I said, shaking my head. Almost immediately, my phone rang. It was journalists. Would I like to comment? Too right I would!

Alfie ran around in delirious excitement as news crews pulled up and set up camp in our dining room. I didn't hold back. Here is an account of one of the news stories on ITV:

'Martin Hibbert, the person closest to the bomb who survived said he was "really disappointed" with the report, calling it "offensive" to the survivors and "even more offensive to those who died".

'Mr Hibbert added that the report offers "no answers" to anything and simply amounted to "people trying to get out of another situation" and "sweep" the issues "under the carpet".

'He added that it "does not come close to the truth", due to "people trying to protect their reputations", who now have "blood on their hands" due to emergency services not entering the arena sooner.

'The forty-one-year-old recalled how "first aiders had to play Roman emperor, they had to say who lived and who died… All they had were first-aid kits and trauma bags" in a scene like "a battlefield from Iraq and Afghanistan".

'He added he "pretty much bled to death on the floor" and believed he was going to die.

'Mr Hibbert, who was at the arena with his daughter, said he was "not going to put up with" the report's findings and if the "truth isn't going to come out by proper means I'll do it myself".'

I was acutely aware that I was a lone voice. I was on my own. Everyone involved in the rescue operation was congratulating themselves for a job well done. To stand up and argue that, actually, what happened was a shitshow wasn't going to make me Mr Popular. I was right. Critics let me have it with both barrels. It stung – of course it did – to read comments like, 'These people did their best – they saved your life' and 'Well, that's gratitude for you!' But I refused to back down. I knew what I'd seen. Heard the cries of people desperate for medical help growing quieter and quieter.

Yes, it was Salman Abedi who had committed this terrible act. He'd planned and set out to kill and maim. But why hadn't he been spotted? And stopped? Why weren't emergency services more prepared? Why were the first-aid kids so inadequate? When people pay a lot of money to attend a public event they expect to be kept safe. To not lose their lives, legs or part of their brain. They don't expect fire crews to turn up more than two hours after the blast happened or for paramedics to be denied access to the site of the blast. I had to speak up. This couldn't happen again. 'I was there,' I insisted. 'I know what happened.' I knew I couldn't have been the only one who felt like that.

I asked Greater Manchester Police to put me in touch with other survivors and families but I heard nothing. 'They don't want us to speak with each other or share information,' I stormed to Gabby.

Then I remembered the Granada documentary and others which had also been screened. I contacted the producers. They agreed to pass my details on to others who had taken part in the programme – both victims of the atrocity and members of the public who had run to help. Responses started trickling through. 'Yes,' they said. 'We'll meet for a chat.'

Five of us met up initially. After cuppas and introductions, I cleared my throat. 'I'm really keen to know what your recollections are of the night,' I began. I wouldn't say a word about my experiences yet. I wanted to hear, first hand, from them.

Robert Grew, who ran to help after hearing the bomb, was one of the first to tell his story. Astonishingly, he now lived just five minutes away from me but, at the time, was living in a flat close to the arena. He'd been in a nearby shop buying food when he heard the explosion. Initially he thought a train had crashed at Victoria Station next door to the arena and ran to see if he could help. Rob is a film producer but also an experienced climber and competent first-aider.

He remembers speaking to a policeman in the NCP car park and asking what had happened. The officer didn't know. As everyone was rushing out of the arena, in terror, Rob ran in. To a scene straight from hell. As far as he knows, the officer stayed outside. Later, he would describe the scene to the official inquiry as 'total and utter carnage'.

'I probably went to you, Martin,' he says now. He remembers a guy kneeling next to me – trying to stop the flow of blood from my neck and keep me calm.

Rob worked solidly and tirelessly until 2 a.m., administering first aid and helping carry casualties down to the assembly point on Victoria Station. Out of consideration for other families and survivors I'm not going to include details of who he treated during those harrowing few hours. He worked with two victims who, sadly, didn't make it, but he treated others who did. Robert was faced with the most horrendous dilemmas: did he stay with the person clinging to him, screaming in pain and terror, or the person who looked like they would need CPR at any moment?

'I just felt incredibly frustrated because there was no help,' he says now. 'Even when I went into the foyer, I was trying to find anything I could use as first aid and there was nothing. We were using torn up T-shirts as tourniquets. Eventually, I found some medical supplies but there was nothing to get people out. We ended up using the signs and stuff from the T-shirt stand and we kind of assembled that and started using the barriers.'

Finally, the last casualty had left the scene in an ambulance. After leaving his details with a GMP officer, Rob had walked the short distance home, alone, stunned, in clothes stained with other people's blood. 'I thought maybe they might be needed for DNA evidence so I kept them in a bag,' he explained. No one ever asked for them.

He rang Greater Manchester Police the next day. They asked him to leave a statement. He wasn't contacted for months – not to clarify anything or for more information. No one asked how he was or offered him counselling: 'I was just this person that turned up and tried to help and then was totally ignored. I didn't know what was going on,' he says. He was relieved now that he was finally in contact with others who had been there. 'I was still trying to figure out what had happened. It was such a chaotic night. I was trying to piece together who I'd helped and if people I'd helped had survived.' It wasn't until September – approximately four months after the bombing – that he was eventually contacted by Greater Manchester Police.

As others told their own, equally shocking, stories, I listened with a growing sense of disbelief, shock, fury and something else. Vindication. I was right. I was bloody right. I hadn't dreamed or imagined the extent of what had gone on and my suspicion that it didn't match the official version was correct. Finally, I told them what had happened to me and Eve. 'We were there for an hour waiting for paramedics to come,' I said. 'I know it was an hour because it was hell having to hang on. I was dying and so was Eve. Twice, she was covered over as people thought she was beyond saving. It's a miracle we survived.'

For a few moments no one spoke. We were all thinking the same thing. Could others who had lost their lives have been saved? Why was no one speaking up about this?

'So what now?' someone said.

'We speak up,' I said determinedly. 'We make our voices heard. The world needs to hear this. What happened was appalling. It can't happen again.'

I offered to organise everything. But it was a mammoth task. I couldn't do it alone. I contacted a friend of mine, Bob Eastwood, an ex-senior police officer and former security and operations manager for the EFL (English Football League) and explained my dilemma. 'I know just the person,' he said. And that's how Andrea Bradbury came into our lives. Apparently he told her, 'I've got a really angry man here who wants to speak with you.' Not only was she a recently retired Lancashire police officer who had served in counter-terrorism, but she and her friend Barbara had been there on the night too – waiting to collect their daughters – and had both suffered leg injuries in the blast.

She and Barbara, now very close, hadn't even known each other that well before the concert. It was their daughters who were friends at drama school. 'We dropped them off at the concert then went for something to eat, as a sort of getting to know you evening and arranged to pick them up later. I didn't even have a clue who Ariana Grande was! I'd retired eight weeks earlier and thought I'd put a frock on and be a lady for the night. I even brought a handbag – I never do handbags.' That bag, worn on her back, took one of the bolts. She is convinced it saved her life.

They were both knocked off their feet by the blast and suffered shrapnel wounds to their legs. Andrea lost consciousness for a couple of minutes. 'There was like an eerie silence,' she says. 'You could see people but there was nothing moving. It was like waking up in some kind of zombie movie.' Eve and I were just a few feet away from her. We were so still, so lifeless, she thought we were dead. 'My priority was getting Barbara to a place of safety.' She says it was like someone had flicked a switch. 'I went from being a friend to being Robocop, shouting instructions. After dragging her out, my next thought was finding the girls. I was pretty sure they hadn't come into the foyer, which wasn't the experience of some mums. I later heard of one woman looking for her daughter among the bodies. She was trying to recognise her shoes and hair.'

Through the cacophony of blaring alarms and Tannoy announcements, Andrea managed to get through to the girls who had fortunately run to a place of safety. She then rang the incident in to the on-call counter-terrorism officer. Andrea's initial assessment was grimmer than the reality, as she guessed thirty were dead. She knew the alarm needed to go right to the top, so, before seeking medical help for her wounds, Andrea hurried straight to Greater Manchester Police HQ to report, first-hand, what she'd seen. She told the inquiry, later, that she was 'left outside' and reported one boss acting like 'a rabbit caught in headlights'. Andrea was an experienced officer. She knew what should have happened on the night. And what didn't.

'It's hard being on the other side,' Andrea says now. 'I've always worked hard in trying to save the public. I've dealt with it all over thirty-one years but nothing, nothing comes close to what happened that night.'

We agreed to work together and formed a support/action group of survivors and families of the bereaved. Andrea came up with the title. 'Survivors Who'll Always Remember Manchester' (SWARM) and threw herself into gathering research. She would conduct detailed telephone interviews, helping them assemble witness statements. She locked herself away in her bedroom while she worked: 'It was so distressing, I couldn't have my family overhearing,' she says.

Meanwhile, I knew we needed legal representation. A firm called Irwin Mitchell was looking after my application to the Criminal Injuries Compensation Authority. All those affected on the night were entitled to apply for compensation. They agreed to represent us. Gradually, others affected heard what we were doing and came forward to join us – relieved that someone was finally listening to them. As a result of our work, some of the survivors were now able to receive mental health support and physiotherapy. Whatever happened now we were stronger together than we were apart.

Ever since 22 May, I'd been staggered at the number of people reaching out to offer support to Eve and me. Old school friends I hadn't seen in years organised a black-tie dinner dance at the Midland Hotel in Manchester, in April. Money raised would go towards any house adaptions needed for Eve and me to cope with our life-changing injuries. They told me they'd secured a VIP guest and when they revealed their identity I thought they were pulling my leg. 'You're joking!' I cried. 'Ron Atkinson?' The manager and player himself. He would be sitting on our top table alongside me and Gabby.

Steve Cook and his wife Louise also came along. And I'd invited a VIP guest of my own: I still had no memory of being treated by paramedic Paul Harvey – but when he arrived I just knew that this man walking towards me, smiling warmly, was him. I'm not sure who reached out first but, simultaneously, we were stretching our arms towards each other. He stooped over, I reached up, and in an instant we were hugging... holding on for dear life. Neither of us spoke. It was all in the embrace. I'd never felt emotion like it. I was too choked to speak. But I hoped he could sense my sentiment. *Thank you. Thank you. Thank you.*

His wife, also called Louise, and Gabby hovered uncertainly for a few seconds – unsure what to do. Then Louise held her arms out to Gabby. 'Shall we have a hug too?' she said tearfully. Paul, Louise and their daughter Scarlett are now close friends.

The night was a resounding success. There wasn't a dry eye in the house as I introduced Paul to everyone as my lifesaver.

A few weeks later, in May, I was over the moon when my Range Rover with hand controls finally arrived. I'd always loved driving and hated being dependent on others to get about. For months I'd relied on Gabby, Mum, my brothers, taxis. Once I'd transferred into the driver's seat, Gabby collapsed my wheelchair and popped it into the boot. 'I'm just going to go around the block a few times,' I said happily as she left and I deeply inhaled that lovely new-car aroma and patted the steering wheel.

Ten minutes later, I was still sat there – frozen with terror. I just couldn't do it. *How can I drive a car without using my feet? What if it suddenly shoots off at 50 m.p.h.?*

Trying not to cry, I rang Gabby. 'Can you come and get my wheelchair out for me, please? I can't do it.' After angrily wheeling myself back inside, I found a driving instructor who specialised in adapted vehicles. On the first lesson, he patiently talked me through the push-pull hand controls which operated accelerating and decelerating. I felt like a seventeen-year-old again as I carefully indicated, checked mirrors and pulled out. 'You can drive, Martin,' he assured me. 'It's just about confidence.'

Within an hour I felt like I'd been driving a hand-controlled car for ever. In fact, I feel far safer using my hands. I feel my reaction times are much quicker. After just one lesson, I drove all the way to Middlesborough to see Karl. 'This is brilliant, Martin,' he said, rubbing his hands. 'Just think of all the good parking spaces we'll get with your blue badge!'

And that wasn't the only set of wheels keeping me occupied. While in the spinal unit, I'd come across a promotion for the Great Manchester Run on 20 May 2018. I'd done a 10k run through Leeds in 2015 and loved it. I watched wheelchair racers go off before the runners, never dreaming I'd be joining them one day. This event would take place just two days before the first anniversary of the attack. I knew the run-up to that time would be incredibly emotional and difficult. A new goal would keep me distracted and motivated. Before I could change my mind, I'd clicked on 'Enter'. There. I had to do it now.

My wheelchair supplier, Cyclone Mobility, put me in touch with Paralympian Richie Powell who agreed to give me some coaching and help me find a suitable set of wheels, as racing chairs are completely different to standard wheelchairs. They still have two large wheels at the back – either side of the seat – but they also have a smaller wheel in front with handheld steering mechanisms.

I tried both kneeling and sitting versions but felt most comfortable in the first. I say, 'comfortable', but racing chairs are designed for speed. Even just getting into it was a challenge. Your bottom sits on the seat with your legs resting on a sloping pad directly below, so you're not sitting directly on your legs.

Richie taught me everything: wedging myself into the 'cage' or seat, crouching low and leaning forwards, to avoid tipping over backwards, something I did many times on my run, leaving me flailing helplessly like an overturned turtle. He helped me master steering and turning the wheels which, believe me, is harder than it looks. Padded rubber gloves provide a really powerful grip on the rubber-coated, push rims on the wheels themselves – enabling you to give a good, strong push each and every time.

However, you don't keep your hands on the rim the entire time. You push three quarters of a revolution, then flick your arms backwards – extending your arms directly behind you, before bringing them forward ready to start the next push.

It took so much practice. There were times I started off pushing too high on the rims causing the front wheel to leave the ground (which was a tad alarming). And hitting a pothole caused every bone in my body to judder. But within a few sessions, I'd mastered the basics. Wheelchair racing requires a huge amount of upper body strength. I didn't have much time to train. But now that I'd committed myself I was determined to see it through. I threw myself into a schedule. Richie, bless him, agreed to race with me on the day. And a good friend Lee Freeman said he'd run alongside us.

Another new friend, Richard Heyes, who had come into my life in the most unexpected of ways, helped me with the training. Richard was a mobile chiropodist and podiatrist who came to the house to tend to my feet. As I couldn't feel them, I was nervous about cutting my toenails, which had grown to resemble an eagle's talons. He was also into health and fitness and started taking me to his gym where he was staggered to see me performing leg curls and extensions on the machines. When I confessed to him that I'd love to go swimming, he rang around every pool until he found one with a hoist – then took me regularly.

A few days before the race, I was invited to the media launch – where I got to meet Sir Mo Farah. I couldn't believe I was being pictured alongside one of our greatest Olympians.

Sunday 20 May was blisteringly hot. A heady combination of nervousness, terror and excitement swirled through my veins. I'd ensured my bowel and bladder preparations were all done in good time. But I still had no idea how my body would respond to race-day nerves or the water I was taking on. Back in 2015, I'd been one of those runners going back and forth to the portaloos, just in case. Today, I didn't have that luxury. The first I knew of needing a wee would be when I realised I'd soaked my pants.

Before the race got underway, a minute's silence descended for the twenty-two victims of the atrocity. It was as if a muffling cloak had been dropped over the thirty thousand competitors and supporters. You could have literally heard a pin drop. Some people were proudly holding up photos of their loved ones. Others waved 'I Love Manchester' signs and placards. I bowed my head and prayed. *There but for the grace of God go I.* This race was for the victims. Every single one of them. Applause rang out from the crowd as the minute finished. Then the iconic Oasis song 'Don't Look Back in Anger' – which has become an anthem of defiance and unity for the city – roared over the speakers.

Waiting for the countdown to start, Richie turned to me. 'Just think where you were this time last year, Martin,' he said. 'You shouldn't even be here.' I nodded. I'd wanted to get around in under an hour but Richie urged me not to put pressure on myself. 'There's no time limit. Just get around and soak it all up.'

Suddenly, there was a honk of starter horns and we were off, speeding through the city centre. The route took us past my beloved Old Trafford and Salford Quays but the scenery was a blur. Instead, I was focusing on a photo I'd stuck to the front of my chair; a photo of me and Eve on my wedding day just four years earlier. She was in her bridesmaid's dress, I was in my morning suit. Looking at that picture as I propelled the wheels gave me a strength and determination I didn't know I had. The muscles in my shoulders, arms and arms burned with effort but I never stopped.

As the finish line and clock on Deansgate came into view, I upped my effort. I could do it. I could beat the hour. My head bowed as I gave the last final push to send me over the finish line. 'Go on, lad!' someone shouted.

'Congratulations to Martin Hibbert!' said the commentator.

I'd done it. 59.07 minutes. It was faster than my previous time of 61 minutes.

I felt slaps on my back. Gabby, my lovely Gabby, appeared. There were cameras everywhere. A reporter crouched down. 'Well done, Martin. How are you feeling?' Five years on, it's still emotional watching the footage. Tears run freely down my face as I answer, 'I'm just really proud. That's for twenty-two people who didn't make it.' On the last two words, my voice cracks and breaks. You can see I'm battling everything to keep the floodgates closed.

'What kept you going?' she asked.

'That picture,' I said, nodding to the photo. 'Hopefully she's watching. The crowd kept me going. I didn't stop all the way round. Not once.' The shrapnel scars on the inside of my left elbow are clearly visible. Sweat and tears plop off my nose as I continue, 'I'm just thinking of when I was in the spinal unit and I couldn't move. Now doing this today…' This time I can't stop the tears. I start to sob and can't stop. Pitifully, I look around for Gabby. The interview is over.

As 22 May 2018 dawned, I was still stiff and sore in my shoulders, back and arms. But it was a good pain. An earned pain. Sipping my cuppa, it felt surreal, listening to news programmes refer to the first anniversary. As I watched the clock, my brain kept thinking back to this time a year ago: I was having breakfast, working at my computer. Life was normal.

At 2 p.m., Gabby and I went to Manchester Cathedral for a service of remembrance for survivors and affected families. Prince William and Prime Minister Theresa May were there along with civic leaders. Police and fire chiefs involved in the response on the night greeted people as they arrived. I couldn't bring myself to shake their hands. Anyone watching might have thought I was churlish. Ungrateful, downright rude even as I fixed my eyes on a point up ahead and, determinedly, kept going. I knew who Eve and I owed our lives to. And it wasn't them.

As we were to learn in the public inquiry, it was thanks to them and the decisions they made that firefighters didn't enter the arena for a full two hours after the bomb went off. It was thanks to them that only three paramedics were ever in the City Room helping the dying and wounded.

Taking deep breaths, I concentrated on the service. Up on the altar, twenty-two pastel-coloured candles were lit. Their flames flickered and danced. We learned during the service that twenty-two brass bees had been added to the cathedral's new choir stalls. The victims would never, ever, be forgotten. The Bishop of Manchester, the Right Reverend Dr David Walker, poignantly told us, 'God has no timetable for our recovery from tragedy. There is no date after which he expects us to have pulled ourselves together. He knows that the hurt we experience can last a lifetime. He is always ready to see our tears, to hear our cries, and to whisper his words of comfort. And you, you who were hurt or bereaved twelve months ago today, are for ever part of Manchester, for ever part of us.'

Gabby's hand crept across and took mine. Once again, my heart swelled with pride at being a Greater Mancunian. At 2.30 p.m. the cathedral observed the national minute's silence. I imagined millions of people bowing their heads, solemnly. Saying a prayer. Wiping a tear. Outside, hundreds were watching the service proceedings on a big screen in nearby Cathedral Gardens. It was also livestreamed at York Minster, Liverpool Metropolitan Cathedral and Glasgow Cathedral.

Afterwards, we emerged into the bright sunlight. I didn't feel strong enough to see the tributes in St Ann's Square. Or to attend a concert there that evening, a performance from the Manchester Survivors Choir. This was a group made up of people who were at the arena that night. Andrea and Barbara were both members – they loved singing their hearts out with others who were there, who understood. I just wanted to be at home. With Gabby and Alfie. My thoughts and my memories.

As the hours ticked by, it became harder to think. To remember. At 6.46 p.m. I had a flashback to the moment Eve and I were smiling for that photo. By 8 p.m. we'd have been walking, excitedly, to the arena. By 8.15 p.m. taking our seats. For two hours we laughed, we sang, we danced, we clinked glasses of Coke. We didn't have a care in the world. As the clock hands inched their way towards 10.30 p.m., I remembered every single second. I saw us, still singing, trotting down the stairs from the VIP boxes, jogging along corridors, entering the City Room. I could see myself reaching out for Eve's hand.

I tried not to think of the CCTV footage of Abedi doubled over with the weight of his deadly rucksack. But it was there. Seared onto my brain.

One second passed. Another. Three... two... one... Then there it was, 10.31 p.m. – the moment our lives, as we'd known them, had ended.

Across the city, bells rang out from buildings. Exactly 365 days, to the very second, since the blast which changed everything. Awful images flashed into my head. I imagined Eve's hand being torn from mine as we were blasted off our feet; hot metal tearing through our flesh like a knife through melted butter.

Sitting there, for the next sixty minutes with my memories and thoughts, I realised an hour is a long time. Especially when blood is pouring from you. And you're scared. Towards midnight and into the early hours, I thought of Mum and Gabby frantically ringing around all the hospitals trying to find myself and Eve; families being given the heartbreaking news that their loved one hadn't made it. As dawn was rising, I took a deep, calming breath. By now, Eve and I were in safe hands. Despite all the odds, we were going to make it.

I thought with a pang how blessed I was. My daughter was still with us. Yes, she'd been left with severe injuries and life would never be the same for her. But she could smile. I could hug her, hold her. Be with her.

Twenty-two other families would take that in a heartbeat.

14

A Growing Anger

May 2018 was a whirlwind – both physically and emotionally. A few days after the first anniversary, I confessed to Gabby that I didn't feel so good. One minute, she was taking my temperature, frowning with concern. The next I was being blue-lighted back to my second home, Salford Royal. Sepsis had got me for the third time in ten months.

As Gabby says now, 'You've had it that many times now that people can get a bit blasé about it. But it's such a dangerous, life-threatening, condition. It terrifies me.'

Sepsis requires prompt treatment with IV antibiotics to tackle the infection that the body has overreacted to. In my case it always stems from a urinary tract infection. Doctors need to identify the exact bacteria causing the infection by carrying out a blood culture test. It can take a few days for results to come back and standard antibiotics are used until specialised ones can be sourced. As a result, it can take a good few days before you even start to turn the corner.

Once I'd started to feel more human, it was lovely to see the nurses, doctors, porters and cleaners who had looked after me a year previously. 'Back again, eh, Martin?' they joked. 'You can't stay away.' I'd been back a number of times to visit them. They were no longer just the medics who had treated me. They were my friends.

My surgeon Mr Saxena, my nurse Stuart Wildman, physiotherapist Caroline Abbott. They have treated thousands of patients over the years but I'm the only one they've formed a close friendship with. Mr Saxena was a bit stunned when I asked if we could meet for breakfast one Saturday morning. I booked a table at George's in Worsley, Manchester. That's now our regular meet-up.

Caroline was a bit wary when I said we wanted to treat her and Stuart to dinner. 'You don't need to, Martin. You've said thank-you.' But I insisted. She sought approval from her bosses to ensure she wasn't breaking any professional rules about socialising with former patients. These amazing people have seen me at the lowest points in my life and have been there, right beside me, at my highest. What happened that night was horrendous. But I treasure the friendships that have resulted.

Most people hate going to hospital and are glad to get out. They might return briefly with cards and chocolates. Then close the door on their way out and keep going. Not me. I love going back to Salford Royal for visits. Every time I see the place, I feel an outpouring of affection, sheer gratitude and love. This place saved me then and has saved me so many times since. No one wants to be ill. But when I am, there's no place I'd rather be.

I returned the first time laden down with gifts for them all. I trundled myself to all the wards I'd stayed on, ITU, HDU, B5 (the trauma ward) and was there for hours – hugging the staff and reminiscing. They were delighted to see how well I was doing. My friends both old and new had been such a support over the last year. I had no idea how I'd ever be able to repay them.

In June, it was my time to step up and be there for Steve. We were watching a World Cup game when I noticed he was a bit quiet. 'You OK, mate?' I asked. He confessed he was concerned about his wife, Suzanne. She hadn't felt well on their recent holiday and had booked a doctor's appointment as soon as she got back. I patted his arm. 'Give over, mate. She'll be fine,' I said. Sadly, I was wrong. A roller-coaster of tests followed. We were all left reeling when Suzanne was diagnosed with cancer. Just three months later, she died.

My heart went out to Steve. Now, I was the one reaching out to him, keeping him going, trying to think of the right things to say. Or saying nothing at all. Just being there and listening. Steve has never been a hugger. But at some point, we started greetings with an embrace. We'd sit and talk for hours. We'd cry together and laugh together.

My therapy and my time with Ken, my long road to recovery, has made me realise the importance of processing emotions. Not bottling them up. Anyone who has seen me being interviewed knows that when the tears come (which they do), I let them flow.

Men are notoriously bad at talking about their feelings and asking for help. Look at me back in 2017, on the very brink of taking my own life. Which is why, in my talks, I started to open up about my mental health struggles. You'd seek a doctor's help for a broken leg or diabetes. Why not depression or anxiety? Afterwards, people started coming up to me and confiding that my words had affected them. They would make an appointment with a medical professional.

I also talk about my wonderful friends. Friendship is the most precious gift in the world. Don't ever take it for granted. Treasure it. Nurture it. I see the little things my friends do, casually pulling up a chair so that we're on the same level. Pointing out a gap in the pavement before my wheel goes into it. And I love them for it. For years, Steve and I had enjoyed going to the cinema, restaurants and clothes shopping in London. Now our trips became more frequent, more important and more difficult – showing just how inaccessible the world can be to disabled people. A step, a flight of stairs, a lift out of order. They all meant the same thing. No entry for those on wheels.

I'd accepted it as just the way life would be. Steve was having none of it. One shopping trip to London stands out in my mind. On visiting a favourite shop, we discovered that menswear was on the first floor. 'Where's your lift?' Steve asked. There wasn't one. We headed across town to the other branch. This time menswear was in the basement. Again, there was no lift. 'We can bring items to you?' a member of staff offered.

'We want to browse,' Steve argued. 'That's the whole point of shopping.' Staff explained the buildings were listed. Lifts couldn't be fitted. 'OK, so why, in just one of your stores, can't menswear be on the ground floor?' he asked. Why indeed. Steve would get so irate on my behalf that I'd have to calm him down.

'It's OK,' I'd begin.

'No, it's not OK, Martin,' he would seethe. 'You're being treated like a second-class citizen.'

We found a Tube station with a lift then took the Underground to Westfield shopping centre in west London. 'Right, I've looked at the map and there's an elevator up to the shops.' Getting my wheelchair on the train was a pantomime. Steve is a strong, fit bloke. He's a personal trainer and goes to the gym twice a day. But he was huffing and puffing to manoeuvre me. 'Gabby would never be able to do this,' he panted. He was right. And that's why we only ever got taxis in London. Which cost us a small fortune.

The elevator was only available from the overground, not the tube station. We were stuck on a platform. The shopping centre was above us. But there was no way of getting up. With a pang I watched everyone else skipping up the steps or stepping onto the escalator. Meanwhile, we had to go back the way we came, to find a tube station with a lift just to get back to street level.

This time, Steve insisted we go to the shopping centre on a bus rather than another train or forking out for a taxi. Buses are far more wheelchair-friendly than tubes or trains. They have ramps that enable you to wheel yourself right on. However, they need to stop first. Steve put his hand out. The driver made no attempt to slow down. In fact, he was speeding up, staring straight ahead. 'He's not stopping,' he said. '*He's not stopping!*'

Steve stepped into the bus's path and put his hand up – forcing the driver to stop, lower the ramp and allow us on. But if Steve hadn't been there, I'd have been left high and dry – watching open-mouthed and helpless as the bus whizzed by. It's little wonder we spend so much time and money in taxis.

Even when lifts are provided in shops and cinemas, there's no guarantee they'll work. I've lost count of the times we've arrived somewhere only to find a dog-eared 'out of order' sign on a lift door. Sometimes, the notice would have been on for months – even years! 'You can't just slap a notice on it and think, Job done!' Steve would fume to staff. He's complained to countless chief executives but nothing ever changes.

Even at some of our favourite restaurants I have to wheel myself in through the fire escape as my wheelchair can't access the steep, narrow entrance. I was shocked to learn that a wheelchair-accessible room, in even a five-star hotel, simply means your wheelchair fits through the door. It doesn't guarantee an accessible shower or facilities, even if you've specified beforehand. I've had more flannel washes than I care to remember, with Steve regularly exasperated on my behalf. 'The guy's in a wheelchair and you've given him a bathtub! How do you think he's going to get into that?'

Then there's the occasions when a too-small cab arrives – after I've specifically requested one I can fit a wheelchair into. I'm often met with a lackadaisical shrug – 'Not my problem'.

After a while, these obstacles do weigh you down. So many able-bodied people don't give them a second thought. Why would they? They're not affected. It doesn't apply to them. However – and I know it's not the most uplifting of thoughts – anyone can become disabled at any time. Believe me, no one chooses to have a spinal cord injury, stroke or motor neurone disease. But these things happen in life. And it's hard enough losing your legs, bowels, bladder and everything else, without additional, insurmountable, obstacles being thrown in your way. 'Every day with an SCI is like climbing a bloody mountain,' I'd sigh, never dreaming how prophetic those words would become.

So, when the Spinal Injuries Association (SIA) asked if I'd consider becoming a trustee of the charity, I didn't hesitate. They had given me so much support and help. Now, it was time for me to give something back. To help others who would be following in my wheelchair tracks, so to speak. I was proud to come on board and vowed to make a difference.

I was also keeping a close eye on the legal proceedings. Inquests into the deaths of the twenty-two victims had opened on 9 June – three weeks after the atrocity – but had been adjourned until after the criminal investigation. The *Manchester Evening News* had reported proceedings had started with a minute's silence for victims from the arena and for those of the terrorist attacks in London: 2017 was a bad year for terrorist attacks, if you remember. We had Westminster Bridge in March, when six people, including the attacker, died and London Bridge in June, when eight people were killed before the three terrorists were shot dead by police.

The coroner revealed on the opening day how nineteen of the arena victims had died at the scene. Three had died in hospital. The inquest also heard how many of those injured had life-changing injuries and a small number had critical injures, including Eve. However, the criminal investigation couldn't get underway until Hashem Abedi, the bomber's brother, had been extradited from Libya. I'd heard how the wheels of justice turned incredibly slowly. Now, I was seeing it for myself.

Various updates trickled through. In autumn 2018, Sir John Saunders was appointed coroner but there was still no prospect of the inquests being held. Meanwhile a parliamentary watchdog of MPs was reviewing all of the 2017 terrorist attacks. I was keen to know what they had to say. In November, the intelligence and security committee reported that MI5 and counter-terrorism police had missed chances to prevent Abedi's attack. I had to take a deep breath before I was able to continue reading.

By now, the media were routinely asking me for comments. 'The truth is now coming out,' I told the BBC. 'It doesn't make things any easier but it means at last there is some compassion being shown and some accountability in terms of people saying, "We didn't do our job." It's a start. It's just sad that it's taken eighteen months.'

Yet the awards to first responders continued to flow. In the Queen's new year honours list gongs were given out like sweets: a British Empire medal, an MBE, a Queen's Police Medal, to various police and fire chiefs who had dealt directly with the attack. 'I can't read any more of this,' I sighed to Gabby. Until now, we'd been receiving updates from the Greater Manchester Police family liaison officer. Now I opted out of the emails.

As 2019 got underway, my diary was fully booked. I'd already arranged my next trip to Australia to see Ken in the summer. I was going to stay longer this time to see what magic might be made. Gabby was going to come initially, then Steve would fly out to join me for a fortnight. The rest of the time I'd be on my own. I lurched between excitement and terror. But, thanks to Ken, my confidence was increasing all the time. 'You can do this, Martin,' I kept telling myself.

Before then was another chance to step out of my comfort zone. 'Skiing?' I asked Gary incredulously. I'd never skied in my life. The thought of doing it now, in a wheelchair, was ridiculous. But he was serious. Teleflex, which makes medical devices like catheters, had teamed up with a sporting activities organisation called Freerider. For sixteen years, they'd arranged an annual ski trip to the Italian Alps for people with SCIs and disabilities. Until now, they'd focused on European countries like Germany and France. But now they wanted to bring it to the UK. After involving Bullen, a healthcare company which worked very closely with the SIA, they decided to run a trial trip. Gary and I had been asked to be the very first participants.

I firmly believe in things happening for a reason and grabbing opportunities – even more so since 22 May. 'Count me in,' I told him. We flew out for the four-day trip in February.

I was a bit apprehensive when I was shown a monoski – a single, wide ski with a seat. Skiing is hard enough on two skis, let alone a single one. But with a bit of practice, and a guide to support me, I quickly got the hang of it. In fact, the only time I fell over was when we were perched in a row, taking instructions. If one person lost their balance, that was it. Down we went like dominoes.

By the end of the first day, my coach agreed I could try a proper run from the top of the hill. Getting up there on a ski lift, seeing the snowy mountainous landscape open out before me, was magnificent enough. But skiing effortlessly down was the stuff of fairy tales. I felt like a bird, flying. The only sound was the soft crunch from my ski as it cut effortless into the fresh, white snow. As I gulped in fresh, Alpine air, tears ran into my goggles. I'm skiing. *I'm skiing!*

It was a relief just to get away from it all. For so long, I'd been organising meetings with survivors and lawyers. Ploughing through paperwork. Doing interviews. In that moment, I was no longer that bloke left paralysed after the arena bombing, that bloke who kicks off over the emergency response. I was just Martin.

The trip still runs every year and I'd encourage anyone with a spinal cord injury to apply. Gary was right. There's no reason why you can't live a full and active life in a wheelchair.

Back at home, the hard work continued. In addition to running my sports management agency, I was working alongside Andrea in speaking with more survivors and families of the bereaved. There was talk of an official investigation being set up. We wanted to be sure we were involved; to get to the truth about what had happened. The second anniversary of the atrocity was also fast approaching. I decided against taking part in the Greater Manchester Run. With the trip to Oz, I couldn't risk overdoing it and succumbing to yet another bout of sepsis.

However, I was honoured to be asked to take part in a promotional mini-film made by the organisers. In 2017, the Great Manchester Run had taken place just days after the bombing. Just before the start, Manchester poet Tony Walsh had read out his poem 'Do Something' – commissioned especially for the event. The words were especially poignant. This year, I was one of a dozen local people – all with inspirational stories – asked to read one line each. My line couldn't have been more apt: 'Do something to make a city proud,' I recited defiantly into the microphone, 'do something to shout, "I will survive".' Our words played against a backdrop of scenes from our amazing city and the run itself.

This year, I wanted to get away from the memorials and media interviews. Instead, Gabby and I flew back to Brisbane to start my second bout of therapy with Ken. My new gym buddy, Richard, also flew out to find out more about NPT. Because of the time difference, I could almost skip 10.31 p.m. on 22 May. I had an emotional hug with Ken and we got straight down to therapy.

Much of our initial work involved easing the spinal lordosis (curve in the lower back) and 'drop foot' (difficulty lifting the front of my feet) that had developed since my last trip. Spending a lot of time in a seated position means it's easy for these niggles to develop. I also had to re-familiarise myself with the tremors required for NPT to work. But within a few weeks I was standing in callipers and building strength in my legs.

My favourite photo from that trip is of me, standing proudly, leaning down to kiss Gabby. One hand is holding the bar. The other is around her shoulders. Her arm is draped around my waist. We were like any other loving couple.

Gabby and Richard had to return for work but Steve flew out in August to keep me company. Every single day he accompanied me to the clinic for my sessions. I made friends with two other lads with spinal cord injuries who were also having treatment. We encouraged each other. I'm still in contact with them, Sam and Alex.

Every day, Steve – now working as a personal trainer – was more astonished at the results. He says now, 'I saw you sitting on those machines, performing a leg extension and leg curl. All I kept thinking was, You shouldn't be doing that... or that.'

We also took some time out for sightseeing – taking a flight to Sydney for a few days. We landed back in Brisbane to learn that my wheelchair had been left behind. 'It will be here in two hours,' they reassured me. They put us in the first-class airport lounge.

That was my first inkling at just how difficult travel can be for people in wheelchairs.

Back on the Gold Coast, we got to know the Uber driver really well on the daily trips to and from the clinic. We talked about everything and anything, including my love of Marvel and Avenger films and one star in particular, Chris Hemsworth. Chris, like his brothers Luke and Liam, had started off in Australian soaps like *Neighbours* and *Home and Away* before making his mark in Hollywood. 'Hey, my friend's dad used to hang out with Chris's dad,' said the driver. 'I'll see if I can arrange for you to meet him.'

Yeah whatever. I'd smile whenever she told me to leave it with her; she was reaching out; working on it. Then one morning, she pulled up – beaming. 'Chris wants to meet you,' she said. 'Can you do this Wednesday?' I waited for the punchline. The 'gotcha' moment. It didn't come. She was looking at me expectantly.

'You're joking,' I said, waiting for the smile to drop. She was serious. I thought of Ken. I had an appointment on Wednesday. 'I'll have to check with Ken. I can't just miss my session.'

When I told Ken, he looked at me incredulously. He actually swore – and Ken never swears. 'What are you fucking asking me for?' he exclaimed. 'He's like royalty. Go!'

As the day drew near, I braced myself for a message. 'Sorry – Chris has got to film.' 'Sorry – Chris has an appointment.' 'Sorry – Chris isn't well.' But it never came. This was happening!

Byron Bay, where he lived, was about a hundred kilometres from the Gold Coast, a stone's throw to Australians. Suddenly, we were pulling up outside his house. He's still incredibly close to family – they all live near to each other – and his dad opened the door. 'He's just at the local radio station, doing an interview but won't be long,' he said. He led us into a huge kitchen. I could feel myself quaking in my chair. *I'm in Chris Hemsworth's house!* Suddenly, the door opened. I swear angels sang as the legend and all-round god that was Chris Hemsworth walked in. All six feet, three inches of him.

'Hey mate,' he called, heading for the kettle. 'Would you like a cup of tea?' He walked towards me – covering the entire kitchen in two casual steps – with his arms outstretched and stooped down and enveloped me in a bear hug. He must have sensed I didn't want to let go, as we stayed like that for ages. Then he hugged Steve.

'You look amazing,' Steve blurted nervously.

Chris grinned. 'You're not looking bad yourself,' he said, keen to know all about his workouts. Steve was on cloud nine.

I switched to full-on stalker mode, gabbling about the films of his that I'd watched over and over and telling him which ones I'd loved (i.e. all of them).

'Hey, we're not here to talk about me,' he said, when he was finally able to get word in. 'I want to hear about you and your amazing story.' He pulled up a chair and listened for more than two hours as I told him all about me and Eve, our injuries and recoveries. I showed him videos of my progress and he said, 'Oh my God, I feel humbled sat here talking to you.'

Before we left, he recorded video messages for Gabby and for Eve. Each starts with me, eyes glittering with excitement, saying to camera, 'There's someone here who wants to say hello.' The camera pans to Chris in all his handsomeness. 'Hey, I'm here with my good friend Martin,' he grins. Eve's message was lovely: 'Me and all the other Avengers wish you all the best,' he said.

Back in the car, Steve and I smiled inanely all the way home. 'Did that really happen?' I kept asking. 'Did we just have a cup of tea with Chris Hemsworth?' The photo of me sitting next to him has become my go-to profile. He really is the loveliest man and we're still in touch today.

The highlight of that trip was still to come, though. I'd been in regular contact with Sarah and Eve throughout my time in Australia. Eve had started at a special school and I loved hearing from Sarah about what she was up to. One afternoon, I opened a video and my mouth fell open in disbelief. The screen went blurry as the tears welled and fell. I picked up the hotel phone and rang Steve. 'You've got to come and see this,' I said.

He burst in and we sat there, side by side, sniffing, as we watched the video over and over. Slowly and painstakingly, Eve had uttered three letters. 'K. F. C.' She had loved takeaways from there. An alert pinged: Mum messaging. 'Eve's started feeding herself!'

I crumpled. Sobbed like a baby. My brave, brave daughter had been to hell and back. But, after two years, here she was, performing miracles. 'I'm so bloody proud,' I wept to Steve. She was on her way. And she'd never look back. I couldn't wait to tell her in person how proud I was of her.

Once again, I was saying my goodbyes to Ken and Nickie and all the other patients I'd made friends with. 'I'll be back before you know it,' I said. I'd realised now that making progression in NPT meant going to Australia as often as I could for as long as I could. It was hard to do it back home without that support network around me.

I was a bit nervous about flying home, alone, but focused on counting down the hours until I saw Eve, Gabby and Mum again. I'd bought myself a lovely lounge suit so that I was ultra-comfy; Calvin Klein joggers and a matching sweatshirt in a stone shade. The airline staff were lovely; they assured me my wheelchair would be well looked-after and wheeled me to my seat in business class. Butterflies fluttered inside me as we took off. I sniffed the air. There was a fragrant, sweet smell. 'Must be curry for dinner,' I thought to myself. But the meal wasn't curry. And even when the plates had been cleared away, the smell was still there.

Sniff sniff.

I shifted in my seat. There it was again. Even stronger. Suddenly, a horrible thought occurred. I went cold. No. Surely not. Oh, please God, no. I glanced down at my new joggers. Praying I was mistaken, I gently eased open the front of my elastic waistband to take a quick peek inside. Then snapped it shut.

Shit.

Shit shit shit.

Yep. And it was *everywhere*.

For half an hour I sat, miserably, biting my nails and stewing in my own excrement. *What do I do? What do I do? What do I do?* I'd sorted my bowels out that morning before leaving for the airport. So, what the heck had gone wrong? Was it nerves? A dicky tum? I had no Gabby or Steve to help. I was now trapped in this seat, at the very front of the plane. For twenty-four hours. You literally couldn't make it up. A bubble of hysteria rose inside of me. I didn't know whether to laugh or cry. Very loudly. Staying put and pretending it hadn't happened was impossible. My skin would break down. Not to mention the torture I'd be inflicting on my fellow passengers.

Eventually, I took a deep breath and pressed the buzzer. An attendant immediately appeared. 'Can I help you, sir?' he asked.

I glanced around nervously, then lowered my voice. 'I'm really sorry,' I said as quietly as I could. 'I've had an... ' My eyes darted to my nether regions, '...accident.'

His expression never changed. He crouched down to keep our conversation private. 'Don't worry about it,' he said, even more quietly than I'd spoken. 'It happens all the time.' *I'm sure it doesn't, but full marks for making me feel better.* 'So, this is what we'll do,' he said. 'We'll turn all the lights down in the cabin. We'll get you into the aisle chair then pop you to the shower room and you can get yourself sorted. And I'll get you some travel pyjamas from first class. How does that sound?'

I nodded gratefully.

This kind, caring, attendant got my bag down from the overhead locker, popped a pair of travel pyjamas inside, then whisked me to the shower room without anyone noticing. It was almost as if he'd flicked an invisibility cloak over me. For the next two hours, I sorted myself out as best as I could with baby wipes. As I opened the door, red-eyed from crying, he appeared from nowhere. 'All good?' he said, kindly, which only set me off again.

Once again, he reassured me it happened all the time. 'Believe you me. Now, I've made you up a new bed here at the back. Get yourself comfy and if you need anything – anything at all, you let me know.'

He and his colleagues looked after me all the way home. They were the epitome of kindness and compassion. I could cry now thinking about that journey. My worst nightmare in the entire world had just happened but I'd survived (which is more than can be said for the Calvin Klein outfit). I often wonder if I'd have got the same treatment on a budget airline...

It felt like I'd been away for ever when I finally touched down at Manchester. Because I'd flown business class, I had a driver waiting to transfer me and my luggage to my car. It would have been impossible on my own. Gabby and Alfie were waiting as I pulled up outside the house. Gabby had festooned banners and balloons to the gate, while Alfie cried and yelped loudly.

'God, I've missed you,' said Gabby, reaching out to to hug me. 'Are you wearing pyjamas?'

'It's a long story,' I replied, rolling my eyes.

Top of my homecoming to-do list was seeing Eve. Nothing prepared me for my daughter greeting me with the words, 'Hi. Daddy.' She spoke slowly, carefully, but she was speaking. So much pride and love surged through me I could hardly breathe. She was doing things we'd never have dreamed of twelve months ago.

The four months away had been a welcome respite from the constant media attention surrounding the atrocity and the aftermath. In July, while I was still away, Hashem Abedi had finally been extradited to the UK to face trial. There was also news from the inquests. In September, Sir John recommended that the inquests should be heard as part of a public inquiry and formally invited the government to set one up.

On 22 October Home Secretary Priti Patel made the announcement we'd all been waiting for. There *would* be a public inquiry. 'It is vital that those who survived or lost loved ones in the Manchester Arena attack get the answers that they need and that we learn the lessons, whatever they may be. This process is an important step for those affected as they look to move on from the attack and I know that they want answers as quickly as possible.'

I read the news with a sense of satisfaction. Finally, finally... we were going to find out what really happened that night. And, this time, I wanted the truth.

15

Fighting Back

As I wheeled myself into Manchester crown court to view the livestreamed trial of Hashem Abedi in February 2020 I realised I was trembling. I'd spent three consecutive nights tossing and turning, desperately chasing sleep that wouldn't come. I was particularly jumpy. I'd never been inside a courtroom before.

I'd done so well since that dreadful night almost three years ago now. I'd carved out a new life for myself. Remained upbeat, positive. I was glad, grateful, to be here. But I was only human. I'd still jump at the boom of fireworks or the slamming of a car door. I'd freeze at the sound of a high-pitched scream. It was only ever a child playing or a toddler having a meltdown in the supermarket but my heart would continue to race for ages afterwards.

I'd feel a wistful pang when Ariana Grande's 'One Last Time' came on the radio. For a moment, I'd be transported back to that VIP box, holding Eve's arms aloft as we swayed. Then the tidal wave would come, engulfing me in a swirling, whirling, torrent of regret, shame, contrition, remorse. Bad/Sad Martin would stir. *Look what you did. How could you?* It would take every ounce of effort to escape his clutches. Break free from the tide of misery – coughing, spluttering and gasping for breath. Desperately, I'd swim for shore. My safe place. My beach. But Bad/Sad Martin was still there in the depths. Waiting to drag me under. There were times when, exhausted and drained, I just needed to give in to the pain.

The bathroom was my sanctuary. I'd turn the shower on full blast. Play music loudly then allow the floodgates to open. I could let it all out, have a bloody good cry, knowing that no one would hear me. I'd weep for Eve and the life she'd lost. I'd weep for the victims and their families. *I'm so sorry that I made it and you didn't.* I'd weep for Gabby, now my carer as well as my wife and for my mum. Finally, I'd emerge – cleansed both physically and emotionally – conscious I'd be doing it all again in a few days' time.

By entering the court I was allowing myself to be taken back to that night. It was terrifying: I had no idea what I'd hear, see and discover over the next few weeks. Whatever I encountered, I knew I wouldn't be able to erase it from my brain. But I'd long made my decision. I'd be there. I had to be. I was grateful that Andrea was beside me, day in, day out. We'd made a deal that we'd attend together. Some of the other survivors and families in our support group didn't feel strong enough to attend. We promised we'd be there on their behalf.

The trial itself was in court two of the Old Bailey, London, livestreamed to courts around the country – including Manchester, Leeds, Glasgow and Newcastle. It was a sombre acknowledgement that people had travelled from all over the country for the concert. Some never made it home again. Others did make it home, but as different people – and that change was also apparent in those close to them who hadn't even been at the show. Not all injuries are visible: Gabby suffered crippling trauma and anxiety as a result of that night. Mid-walk with Alfie, she'd find herself seized by terror, gripped by an all-consuming panic that a terrorist was lying in wait in their car, planning to mount the pavement and mow her down. Thousands of people were left scarred in some way by what Abedi unleashed that night. And, as we were about to learn, he didn't act alone.

In the long run-up to this day, there had been times I wondered if the trial was worth it. The bomber had been obliterated by his own bomb. His younger brother wasn't even in the country. How could he have been involved? But by the end of the three-week process, there was no doubt. Hashem Abedi was just as guilty of murder as his brother. I'd wanted to see him in the dock, but he had the privilege of being shielded by a screen and missed so many days; his legal team pleaded ill health, dehydration (allergic to tap water, apparently), tiredness, difficulty concentrating, the court day being overly long, Abedi being overwhelmed with the whole process and suffering flashbacks. You really couldn't make it up. Other days there was no reason given, he just refused to leave his cell. On day twenty-four, his QC told the judge Abedi 'no longer wished to participate in the trial'. And two days later, he sacked his entire legal team.

He must have known it was over. Over the course of the trial, we heard compelling evidence that Hashem had been involved with his brother in ordering, stockpiling and transporting deadly materials to create the bomb. The jury deliberated for just three and a half hours. The name of each victim was read out. The verdict the same. Guilty. The one count of attempted murder (relating to all those who had been injured but survived) and one count of conspiracy to cause an explosion: guilty. Thank God.

Afterwards Assistant Chief Constable Russ Jackson of Greater Manchester Police said that Hashem Abedi was 'every bit as guilty as his dead brother. He was his brother's driver, the quartermaster sourcing deadly material and the munitions technician in those months running up to the attack'.

As the trial had progressed into March 2020, the news had become more dominated by the early stages of the Coronavirus pandemic. It began to affect proceedings. One of the jurors became ill and had to self-isolate. Just six days after the verdict we entered the first lockdown. The judiciary system – like everything else in the country – ground to a halt. Abedi's sentencing was put back until August. Andrea and I had planned to be at the Old Bailey in person. I'd wanted to wheel myself in there defiantly and show him he hadn't won. But with Abedi refusing to attend there was little point. I publicly backed the campaign to make it compulsory for convicted criminals to be present at sentencing.

Instead, I watched the outcome on TV, nodding with satisfaction on learning that trial judge Mr Justice Baker had sentenced Abedi to fifty-five years in prison. 'The stark reality is that these were atrocious crimes: large in their scale, deadly in their intent, and appalling in their consequences,' he said. He told the court how he had read 'many' victim impact statements, including the one I'd submitted on behalf of Eve and me, concerning lives either 'extinguished or forever blighted.' 'Many of the survivors have explained their feelings of enduring guilt and shame at having survived these dreadful events.' So, it wasn't just me. 'However human these feelings may be, I hope that in time they may be able to accept that the only individual who should have any such feelings is the defendant whose actions, together with those of his brother, were entirely responsible for those events.'

Throughout the spring and summer of 2020, Andrea and I, along with other members of the support group, had been battling for our voices to be heard at the forthcoming inquiry. Back in October, Sir John had invited applications for 'core participant status' – people who would play a key role in the inquiry.

Having only recently returned from Australia, I was spending time with Eve, catching up on medical appointments and trying to run my business. We were all still having treatment for injuries – both physical and mental. Before we knew it the deadline had passed. Our own solicitors Irwin Mitchell submitted a late application on behalf of a total of fifty-six survivors, including me, Eve and Andrea. With the country now in lockdown, proceedings were carried out virtually. On 21 April, Sir John announced his decision: no. He argued that the terms of reference of the inquiry focused on those who had lost their lives rather than those who had survived. Our legal team asked him to reconsider, but it was still no.

Ever hopeful, we applied for a judicial review of the decision. We lived and breathed our application, poring over submissions and legal papers to get it right. Over two full days, on 8 and 9 July, we followed proceedings online. We had all submitted our own statements and our barrister did a great job in putting our case forward.

On 29 July we heard the result. Sir John declared that we would get to 'contribute to and engage with' the inquiry as witnesses. We could attend hearings, watch via livestream, access transcripts, evidence and documents on the website, raise issues, suggest lines of questioning... but, no, we would not be granted core participant status.

'I hope that this decision is not too much of a disappointment to survivors,' he said. 'As I have said at the outset, the survivors clearly have significant evidence to contribute and I invite them to assist me as witnesses. They will be provided with the necessary disclosure relevant to their accounts to enable them to do this effectively and I would ask them to provide me with any insights and observations that they have so that they can be investigated in so far as they come within the terms of reference. He concluded, 'Their voice is an important one and it will be heard.'

We made a last-ditch attempt to take it to the European Court of Human Rights, where it was turned down. Reluctantly, we agreed we'd done all we could. So that was that.

Our application had been made with the best of intentions. We had no wish to tread on anyone's toes. We simply wanted to ensure our voices were heard. We were the only people who saw, first-hand, what happened that night. The victims no longer had a voice. And many of the bereaved families hadn't been there. We genuinely thought we could play a valuable part. Dejected, I turned my back on the inquiry. When I was asked if I'd consider giving evidence as a witness, I fumed, 'They must be joking! They turned us down when we wanted our voices heard. Now they want me to give evidence? No. I bloody well won't.' Yes, I was being a dick. But after all we'd gone through, I was feeling sore and slighted. My statement, on behalf and Eve and myself, was submitted. And that, as far as I was concerned, was it. The inquiry would conclude in March 2023.

In the spring of 2020, as the third anniversary of the bombing approached, once again, I looked for something else to focus on. A goal to keep me busy. A few months earlier, Gary had had the perfect idea. Each year the SIA ran an international cycling event to raise funds. This year they'd be cycling across northern Italy on handbikes. Brilliant. I signed up. Threw myself into training, only to be gutted when the coronavirus meant the trip was put on hold. And then an idea formed. We couldn't go to Italy. But Italy could come to us!

We each got hold of a turbo trainer, which transforms any ordinary bike into a stationary training bike, then agreed we'd do the first stage – a sixty-six-mile challenge around Tuscany – simultaneously from our living rooms in lockdown. We encouraged others to sponsor us or join 'Gary and Martin's Virtual Cycle Italia' event. Our bikes were set up with the gradients we'd have been tackling to match every real hill and steep climb.

On the morning of 14 May, we set off, livestreaming our efforts. We appeared on *BBC Breakfast* news, local radio and TV, puffing and panting as we answered questions while cycling. There was no lovely scenery or cheering crowds to keep us going – just my ceiling. And I had the added challenge of Alfie randomly choosing to sit on me and lick my face. My arms were on fire as we approached the virtual finish line and I was ready to collapse as I posted the final clip on social media.

I was touched when lawyers from Irwin Mitchell, the legal firm representing us, also joined in remotely. In total, we raised sixteen thousand pounds. It was a drop in the ocean compared to what was needed: the SIA had taken a huge knock during Covid-19. Not only were no funds being raised but reserves were being gobbled up at an alarming rate. There had never been so little money in the pot and so much demand. The support teams and helpline were run off their feet. 'We need to come up with a really bonkers idea to get money coming in,' I suggested to Gary during one of our Zooms. 'I'll get thinking.'

This year's anniversary under lockdown conditions would be incredibly different. There would be no memorial service. No visit to Eve or laying of flowers. I was secretly pleased when *The Morning Show* on 7News in Australia asked if they could do a live interview with me about the NPT therapy I'd had with Ken and the virtual cycle challenge I'd just completed. I stayed up late so I could appear and, suddenly, I was being beamed into living rooms all over Australia. We had a lovely chat for ten minutes. Then they finished by announcing they had a special message for me. Suddenly, Chris Hemsworth filled the screen. 'Hey there, Martin,' he grinned. 'Hope you're doing well buddy. Just wanted to say the time that we spent together in Australia was truly inspiring, mate. To meet someone who had faced such adversity and such dramatic challenges… but to see someone like yourself with such a positive attitude was incredible, mate. To face that road to recovery with such determination and commitment is absolutely inspiring. You're one of a kind, and I can't wait to see you soon as we walk down the red carpet together, mate. Be well, stay strong. And see you soon.'

Bloody hell. Not only had Chris Hemsworth remembered me. He'd invited me to walk down the red carpet with him. I didn't know whether to laugh or cry. 'Thank you,' I told them, clearly emotional. 'You don't know what means.'

Thanks to Zoom and Teams I could still work and even keep doing my inspirational talks. Bosses were keen to keep their staff motivated and inspired through the pandemic. During the summer I spoke with members of Pro-Manchester, a business development network. I had no idea how many were tuning in but got some lovely messages in the comments box. Looking back now, I'd forgotten how isolated everyone was. Just seeing another face or hearing another voice, made the world of difference.

Room54, a bureau of professional speakers, got in contact to suggest I take up public speaking professionally. Their boss, Layla Jenkins, liked one of my speeches. My initial response was to laugh. Martin Hibbert from Bolton? A public speaker. Don't be ridiculous. But she assured me that people wanted to hear my story. She'd heard the reactions. *Uplifting. Inspiring. Heartbreaking.* Also, wasn't it one in the eye for the terrorists? Telling the world that they'd never win. We'd come back stronger. I could promote awareness of living with an SCI, talk about living with depression.

'OK,' I said. 'I'll do it.' As bookings arrived, I remembered, with a wry smile, all the tellings-off at school; all the teachers who'd said I might do well in life if I could just, occasionally, *shut up!* Motivational speaking is now my full-time job. I love it.

Throughout that first lockdown, I'd been so cautious when it came to my health. Not only did I need to keep covid at bay. But with all medical appointments cancelled for the foreseeable, I had to be ultra-careful about everything involving my skin, bowel and, in particular, my bladder. People with SCIs are particularly prone to urinary tract infections. And I was more prone than most, as I was about to discover. I emptied my bladder regularly. Drank lots of water. Monitored my output. Washed my hands scrupulously. Did all the right things until, one night in July, I woke feeling hot and shivery. I rang Gabby on her mobile. 'I don't feel well,' I slurred. My temperature was through the roof. Within minutes, I was being blue-lighted to hospital.

Here we go again...

This time was grimmer than usual, for countless reasons. Instead of being taken to Salford, where they all knew me, I went to another hospital. Covid regulations meant Gabby couldn't visit, let alone come in with me. I couldn't bring my wheelchair. And the hospital was overrun and desperately short of staff.

As all the beds were full, I was admitted to a makeshift ward and set up with IV antibiotics while waiting for blood cultures results to come back. Before covid, I had developed a routine in hospital with my infections because I'd had so many: a nurse would insert an in-dwelling catheter to drain off urine and place a fan by my bedside to cool me down. They'd then monitor my vitals and keep on top of medication while, reassured and feeling safe, I'd slip into repairing, healing sleep.

This time was different. The bed and mattress weren't suitable for a patient with an SCI. Fretting about pressure sores, I had to continually change my position. I was continually leaking urine, due to the raging infection in my urinary tract, but staff did not insert a catheter. My pyjamas were constantly soaked. I was terrified of my skin breaking down. An in-dwelling catheter would solve the problem at a stroke.

'We'll get you sorted,' someone would say. But I'd never see them again.

The time for the medication trolley appearing would come and go without any sign of it. Occasionally, someone would appear to take my temperature. 'Ooh,' they'd say, raising their eyebrows. 'It's gone up again.' Eventually, I couldn't hold back. 'No shit, Sherlock! Maybe it's because I haven't had my medication or a catheter fitted.' The nurse bristled. 'You can't talk to me like that,' she said. But it was true.

As time passed, my annoyance turned to anxiety and then cold fear. One evening was particularly bad. I pressed the buzzer. No one answered. The other patients took pity on this poor, paralysed man crying in his bed and they pressed their buzzers as well. Still, no one came. In desperation, I rang Gabby. 'I'm going to die here, on this ward,' I said. 'Please, please come and get me.' She calmed me down. Assured me she'd contact the hospital. I lay there listening to the ward phone, out in the corridor, plaintively ringing. No one answered.

In desperation, Gabby rang the chief executive of the SIA, who rang the chair, who alerted Gary, who tried a nurse he knew. They were all ringing the ward, saying I urgently needed attention to prevent complications. No one answered. My prayers were only answered when a lovely ward nurse happened to come on shift. 'How are you getting on, Martin?' she asked kindly.

I burst into tears. 'I've never been so scared,' I confessed. 'Even on the floor of the arena, when I was dying, I wasn't this frightened.'

She was truly horrified. 'I'm so sorry, Martin,' she said, shaking her head. 'This is awful. I can't apologise enough.'

I reached out for her hand. 'Please,' I begged. 'I just want to go home. I don't feel safe here. At least at home, I've got my wheelchair and my shower chair so I can go to the toilet. I've got Gabby to look after me.' Although my infection markers were still high, doctors agreed I could be discharged with my antibiotic medication in tablet form. When Gabby brought me home, I was so weak that I couldn't even transfer from the car to my wheelchair. Mike, our dog carer, was dropping Alfie back at the same time. He had to scoop me out of the car and carry me into the house.

I have never been so relieved to be in my own bed. I spent two weeks there recovering. And thinking. This was wrong. I'm a bolshy, outspoken bugger, well able to speak up, stand up for myself. If *I* felt like that on a hospital ward, how would others with an SCI fare? People with this type of injury can't just hop out of bed and shuffle off in search of a nurse. They are stuck. That scenario could be being repeated in hospitals and care homes up and down the country. We'd heard nightmare stories of people contacting the helpline in desperation. Carers had stopped attending. These patients were absolutely stranded. Alone. Terrified.

Once I felt stronger, I was able to attend virtual meetings with the charity again. The mood was grim. We were in financial dire straits. Those higher up estimated that, by the end of the pandemic, we'd be down a million pounds in lost donations. 'Right, what can I do to raise that?' I asked. 'It's got to be something hard. Something that will make people sit up and think, He's doing *what?* Something that will make people dig into their pockets to sponsor me.' Suddenly, I remembered what I'd said before about the battles people with SCIs had, that they climb a mountain every single day. 'Why don't I climb Everest?'

Silence.

I looked around the screen at their expressions – from bemused, confused ('What did he say? My screen froze') to perplexed. 'It's impossible,' someone finally said.

'OK, not Everest,' I conceded, 'but what mountain could I do?'

Brows furrowed as people thought of, then dismissed, the world's most dangerous peaks... K2, Mont Blanc. Then someone mentioned Kilimanjaro in Tanzania. Not only was it the world's highest free-standing mountain (meaning it wasn't part of a range) – it was the highest mountain in Africa and one of the famous 'seven summits', the highest peaks of each of the seven continents. Karl had climbed it twice. It was doable, surely? 'So, I'll do that,' I announced. My voice was getting faster and higher as I ran away with the idea. 'I can put a team together. Let's challenge this notion that disabled people can't do these things. We'll turn an appalling act of terrorism into something positive. Bring people together in a spirit of hope. I'll involve the very people who saved my life that night.'

There was silence again. But no one said 'No' this time. I knew what they were all thinking: logistics, health and safety, risk assessment, costs. 'Look, I'll do it. I'll make it work,' I vowed. I was flushed with excitement by the time I signed off. Immediately, I googled 'how hard is to climb Kilimanjaro?' The positivity balloon that had been bobbing cheerfully above my head deflated noisily as I read that the odds of success were only 65 per cent. And that was for an able-bodied person. For a few seconds, I was crushed. And then I remembered Grandad's words. 'Don't wait for your ship to come in, Martin, lad. Go out and meet it.'

I also recalled my conviction, my overwhelming belief, that Eve and I had been saved for a reason that night. 'I don't know why, yet, but I'm sure I'll find out,' I'd said in countless interviews. So, was this it? Was this why I'd survived? Flexing my fingers, I opened a new email and cc'd everyone from the board of trustees. In the subject line I typed two words: 'Martin's Mountain'.

Bring it on.

16

A Bonkers Idea

'Next time you have a bright idea, Martin Hibbert, keep your gob shut!': that was Gabby's response when she realised what I was up to.

She was used to hearing my continual chatter on Zoom calls – whether for work or my involvement with the SIA. Mostly it went over her head. But she stopped dead walking through our dining room one day just as I was uttering the infamous words: 'Look – to raise a million pounds, it needs to be something I risk my life for – otherwise it's not worth it.'

I finished the call to find her standing there. 'What are you up to?' she asked.

'Climbing Kilimanjaro,' I beamed.

In one instant, ten different expressions flashed over her face. Laughter (not for long), disbelief, shock, anger, worry: 'After everything you've been through, Martin, why would you want to put yourself through this?'

It was hard to explain. But this was something I had to do. By some miracle, I'd survived that night. I'd been given my life back. Now, I had a duty to give back to the charity that had got me here. Besides, I wasn't doing it on my own. The whole point of the expedition was to show that, with the right team and support, anything was possible. 'It'll be fine, love, I promise.'

Gabby didn't look overly convinced. But she knows more than anyone how any attempt to change my mind on anything only makes me more determined to do it.

Besides, the plans were well underway. Through reaching out to expedition experts, we'd discovered that climbing Kilimanjaro in a wheelchair was an 'exceptional feat' but could be done. However, I'd need a crack team.

'Caroline and Stuart,' we agreed. It wasn't just because they were among our closest friends now. Or that they'd seen me at my lowest, so deserved to see me at my best. I also wanted to shift attention away from the atrocity. I wanted the focus to be on the people who had helped me adapt to life in a wheelchair, not those who had put me in it. But – and it was a huge 'but' – it was a massive undertaking, involving months of arduous training and the best part of a fortnight in Africa. What if my potential team said no? Oh God, what if *everyone* said no? But Caroline didn't even let me finish my question before answering. 'Absolutely,' she'd cried.

Now, I just had to persuade Stuart. He had a young family and might not be so keen. Just as I'd done when I was a child rehearsing comebacks to neighbours who didn't want their car washed, I practised what I'd say beforehand. I spent a weekend listing all the reasons why he'd be mad not to take up this incredible opportunity, before ringing him on the Sunday morning while he was having his coffee in bed.

Here's how the conversation went: 'Hi Stuart.'

'Hi Martin. How are you?'

'I'm good, thanks. Listen, I need to ask a favour.'

'Yep, anything.'

'I'm climbing Kilimanjaro and I'd like you to do it with me.'

'Yep, no problem.'

There wasn't even the slightest hesitation. 'Bloody hell, Stuart,' I cried. 'I've spent a weekend planning how to talk you round.'

He's told me since, 'I didn't even have to hesitate. The "Yes" came from inside. All I could think was, What an honour,' although he admits that he'd turned to his wife and asked, 'What have I just agreed to?'

An old friend, Mark Pilling, from my Barclays days, got in touch. 'Hey Martin, I quite fancy doing this climb with you,' he said.

'Get on board, man!' I told him, delighted.

I was touched by his fundraising message: 'I still recall, to this day, the anguish of the one tick on WhatsApp when I asked: "Martin, is all OK?" Fast-forward four years and Martin has achieved more than I think he ever felt possible. I'm inspired by him every day. I'm determined to help Martin raise the million pounds and will be so proud when he does reach this target because he will! If you know him, you know he won't stop.' And that was the sort of encouragement I needed to hear.

I also wanted my best friends at my side. Karl, a seasoned climber, promised to support me but said, and I quote, wild horses wouldn't get him up there for a third time. However, he gave me so much advice and encouragement that it was like having him there.

The trip was scheduled for September 2021 and would coincide with the third anniversary of losing Suzanne. But assured by his family that she would want him to do it, Steve signed up.

Rob Grew, who had raced into the arena to help, was not only a good friend by now but an experienced mountain climber so I was chuffed when he said he'd be glad to join in.

Ollie Buncombe, SIA's challenge events coordinator and his wife Nadia, were also on board.

The ninth slot went to Graeme Hackland, chief information officer at the Formula One team Williams Racing. The late team boss, Sir Frank Williams, had suffered a spinal cord injury after a car crash in 1986 and the SIA has been the team's official charity since 2015.

The tenth member would play a crucial role. In fact, the success of the trip depended on them. Climbing a mountain is hard enough for an able-bodied person. Throw in a spinal cord injury and you open up a whole new catalogue of health risks and worries. Believe me, not being able to walk is the least of your worries. Less movement in my body – from the point of injury downwards – means poorer blood circulation. This affects temperature control. If I get cold, it's harder to warm up. I can't feel my legs or feet. There's also a risk of swelling, or oedema, in the legs. Any skin chafing could lead to a blister or sore which could lead to skin breakdown and infection and that's without the whole bladder and bowel shenanigans. The icing on the cake was the 'S' word: sepsis. If sepsis took hold, it was game over, not just for my challenge but, potentially, for me as well. This meant I'd need a nurse on hand, one specialising in spinal cord injuries, to be at my side, day and night. It would be a huge responsibility and I will forever be indebted to Chris Paton for stepping up.

Chris responded to an appeal from the SIA. But he had a whole list of questions that we needed to answer before committing. He explains, 'Skin, bladder and bowel are the three biggest problems for someone with an SCI. In an alien environment things can get difficult. And any difficulties would be firmly on my shoulders.' He wanted to be assured of my base level of health and fitness, my history of pressure sores or skin breakdowns and he needed to know if I'd be sitting on any of my scars or old wounds. He also had to be given details of my bowel and bladder regime.

Intermittent catheterisation would be too difficult going up a mountain, he decided. I'd need to use an in-dwelling catheter, silver-coated to reduce the risk of infection, with the bag emptied regularly. 'A measurable volume coming out means I can also keep an eye on your water intake,' he explained. Enemas would also be difficult so I'd have to master emptying my bowel a different way.

Allow me to introduce you to digital stimulation: a 'digit' is a finger. And stimulation is, well, stimulation. Put the two together and what have you got? That's right. A finger up the back passage. As with the enema, you prepare with a laxative the night before and a suppository an hour earlier. Then, wearing a medical glove and using lubrication, you lie on your left-hand side, in the foetal position, insert your index finger up your back passage, and move it in a figure of eight pattern. This stimulates the bowel, encouraging the poo to move into the lower part of the rectum where it can be evacuated. Although Chris would perform the honours on the trek I had to train my bowel and body to respond to this new technique.

Kilimanjaro doesn't call for any technical mountaineering but it is still a tough challenge so we'd all need a good level of fitness. We'd follow personalised training programmes and also undergo altitude and cryotherapy training – that's using cold to boost muscle recovery and improve performance.

For the logistics of the trip, we partnered with AdAstra Adventures, run by Kat Shrives, whose mum Katy suffered an SCI in a riding accident when Kat was twelve. The date was set for September 2021, to coincide with the covid-delayed Paralympics in Tokyo.

Most climbs ascend from the south of Kilimanjaro. But AdAstra decided our route to the summit would go via the Rongai route from the north. 'It's quieter but also has much easier terrain on the ascent and you have less altitude gains each day,' Kat explained. 'Others who have summited in wheelchairs have all used this route.'

The forty-five-mile ascent would take approximately five days, with three days for the descent, taking in rainforests, boulder fields, sand dunes, slippery volcanic slopes, and snowy peaks. We'd have one of the best teams of local guides, trek doctors and porters. They'd prepare our camps each night and ensure we stayed safe and well.

On the actual ascent, the focus would be on gradual acclimatisation under continuous monitoring by expedition leaders and medics. In particular, they'd be looking out for signs of altitude sickness – a lack of oxygen to the tissues and, most importantly, the brain, caused by exposure to low air pressure.

Symptoms include headaches, excessive fatigue, nausea/vomiting and dizziness. Early symptoms, we learned, can be overcome by staying hydrated, nourished, well rested and by ascending gradually. However, altitude sickness isn't something you can control or push on through. It has nothing to do with your abilities and fitness levels. It affects everyone in different ways. In severe cases, it can be life-threatening. If we felt ourselves succumbing, it was important to speak up immediately and seek medical help. It usually resulted in the affected person being taken back down the mountain as quickly as possible. The summit would have to wait. But at least you'd be safe.

My team also needed to be trained in manual handling to ensure they were confident in lifting me and my wheelchair over boulders and crevices. We put all our skills and kit to the test on training camps around the UK so that nothing was left to chance. As the months passed, it all started coming together. I'd be ascending in a custom-built, specially adapted mountain trike designed for tackling mountainous terrain.

Peter Hutchinson Designs (PHD) created specialist expedition clothing for me – including salopettes, socks and booties to keep my feet warm at night – all with carefully repositioned zips to guard against irritation and pressure sores.

The team bonded over our preparation sessions. The altitude training involved actual physical workouts on spin bikes or on SkiErg training machines, exercising while fitness professionals analysed our blood oxygen levels. If we dropped below a certain point we were asked to leave the room to recover. We'd take bets on who would be kicked out each week. I'm delighted to say it was never me!

We also endured cryotherapy training at Burnley College to boost our immune systems and aid our recovery. We'd wear minimal clothing but don specialist kit like gloves, earmuffs and headbands to protect the extremities. On entering the chamber you'd brace yourself as the temperature dropped to minus ninety over three minutes. It was absolutely freezing but you felt great afterwards. And no matter how gruelling the training, I'd wake up each morning fresh and raring to go. 'I feel like bloody Superman,' I told Gabby.

I was starting to look like Superman, too. Pretty soon my work shirts were straining at the shoulders. 'Look at these guns,' I'd say to Gabby, flexing my biceps.

As word spread, reactions varied from disbelief and encouragement (most people) to terror (me mum) and humour (from my brother Andy). 'You've never climbed so much as a bloody ladder!' he chortled, 'and now you're climbing a mountain?' He was right. The old Martin would never have taken on something like this in a million years. But the attack had changed me in so many ways.

Meanwhile, in April 2021, the inquiry was well underway. I went along to support Andrea as she appeared as a witness but was still adamant I wasn't taking part. Then the counsel to the inquiry, Paul Greaney QC (now KC), asked to see me. 'We've got your statement, Mr Hibbert, but the chairman Sir John Saunders would really like you to consider being a witness.' My statement had confirmed that I was one of the few people, still conscious, for almost an hour in that room, waiting for help. My participation could really make a difference to the inquiry. Finally, I agreed, but I told them I'd like something in return.

I wanted to see what happened to me and Eve before, during and after the bomb went off. My request was greeted with silence. Then Paul Greaney replied. He wasn't sure it was a good idea. I interrupted. 'I see what happened in that arena every single night before I go to sleep. I'm not seeing anything I haven't seen before. It will just really help me process and make sense of what happened.' He assured me he'd look into it.

In May 2021, the Kilimanjaro team set off on our first training expedition up Pen y Fan in South Wales, a 2,906-foot peak. 'It's been gruelling, it's been frustrating at times, but we've got to the top and the views are absolutely spectacular,' I said as I smiled to camera. It was nothing compared to Kilimanjaro at 19,000 feet, but it was a start.

As the summer progressed, it was clear that covid was still very prevalent. With a mixture of disappointment and relief at having more time to prepare, we postponed the trip to the following June. One member of the team was delighted. In early 2021, Caroline had discovered she was expecting and thought she'd have to drop out. But the change in date meant she could take part after all. After her daughter Grace was born in July 2021, Caroline threw herself back into training.

A few days later, I heard back from the inquiry. GMP had agreed to me viewing material from the night. Steve was allowed to come. He wouldn't be permitted to look at anything but I just wanted him in the room. Seeing those images from CCTV and bodycam was like stepping back to a different world. There were black-and-white shots of Eve and I walking through the City Room on the way to the arena. Walking. Something we'd both taken for granted. She'd have been excited. At one point she was hugging my arm, looking up at me, smiling.

At 10.30 p.m., there we were again – heading back into the City Room. In those images, we were frozen in time. Another life. Another world. There were people all around us. Some, like us, were walking quickly towards the car park doors. Others were leaning against pillars, watching the doors closely for the first glimpse of their teenagers emerging from the concert. I gazed at them. How could any of us have imagined what was about to happen?

Another black-and-white picture showed us one second before detonation. Abedi was just out of sight. The officer paused with his hand on the file. 'Before I turn this over, I need to say that the next image is post-detonation. Are you sure you're ready for this?'

I took a deep breath. 'Thank you, but I'd like to see them.'

My hands were trembling now. He nodded. 'If you need to stop at any time...'

His fingers took a corner of the photograph. And turned it over.

Instinctively, I flinched. And there it was. The City Room after the explosion. There I was, in my jumper and jeans, lying motionless, in a pool of blood. Eve was just out of sight but other images showed she was no more than a few metres away from me. Everyone around us was dead. Another image showed the security guard crouched down, trying to stop the bleeding from my neck. But the angle of my head never changes. My eyes are open. Trained on Eve. Fixated on her.

Other people come and go in the images that followed. I bristled as I saw Eve, twice, covered over with a white poster. I remembered desperately trying to alert first-aiders to the fact she was still alive. Still breathing. I could almost feel the blood gargling in my throat as I relived those moments. More pictures were turned over. All this time, I'd convinced myself Eve was carried out first. I can remember telling myself, 'She's safe. You can go now,' as I slipped away. I was staggered to see that, actually, I'd left the City Room before she did. I'd lost so much blood by that point, it's not surprising I was confused. But why did that happen?

I found comfort knowing we were never more than ten metres apart at any time, in the casualty clearing area at Victoria Station, waiting for ambulances. I wondered if she sensed me there. Urging her to hang on. Finally, we'd reached the last grainy image. We were done.

I exhaled shakily. 'Thank you,' I said. 'It's really helped.'

Yes, those images were horrific. The majority of survivors and bereaved families wouldn't benefit from seeing them. But it was something I needed to do. For four years, I'd been tortured by my memories and dreams. But those images confirmed I'd looked out for my daughter. Kept her safe. Just like I'd promised when I held her in my arms as a newborn.

She wasn't on her own. Daddy was there. I felt a strange sense of peace. I was ready to testify.

In the meantime, the first report from the inquiry was about to be published.

Sir John had already announced that the first report would focus on the security arrangements on the night, the second would concentrate on the response of the emergency services and the third would look at intelligence. As the date drew nearer, I became more anxious. Would it be a whitewash? Would I be as disappointed as I had been with the Kerslake report? Would I, once again, have to shout to be heard?

Finally, the report was launched. 'I have concluded that there were serious shortcomings in the security provided by those organisations which had responsibility for it and also failings and mistakes by some individuals,' Sir John announced. I exhaled a long, deep, sigh of relief. Finally, we were getting somewhere. The truth was coming out. ' ... There were a number of opportunities to identify Salman Abedi's activities as being suspicious on the night before he detonated his bomb. What I cannot say with any certainty is what would have happened if those opportunities had not been missed.'

The report revealed that Salman Abedi had returned from Libya four days before his attack. He spent that time putting the finishing touches to the bomb that he and his brother had been working on for months and making three 'hostile reconnaissance' visits to the City Room. He'd watched queues of ticket buyers and sought out blind spots in the City Room that were not covered by CCTV or routinely patrolled by security guards. This grim knowledge enabled him to loiter on the night undetected for two hours before detonating his device.

While Eve, I and 14,000 others had been having the time of our lives in the Arena itself, he'd been skulking and shuffling back and forth between the City Room and Victoria Station. It was a warm evening and he was overdressed, stooped over by the weight of the deadly plus 30-kg load on his back.

CCTV images showed him walking slowly past two members of the security staff who were wearing high-vis vests and two

BTP Police Community Support Officers (PCSOs). At 8.51 p.m. a security guard on duty in the City Room did notice Abedi enter. He remembered liking the trainers Abedi was wearing and noticed he was wearing a camping rucksack. But no alarm bells rang. Abedi left twenty minutes later, returning again at 9.30 p.m. Again, the same security guard saw him. This time, Abedi walked up the stairs to the mezzanine or upper level area of the foyer and sat down out of sight, leaning against a wall.

Biding his time.

Waiting.

Five BTP officers should have been on duty that night. One, the most senior, did not attend until after the explosion. Of the four who were on duty, three were PCSOs. They had been told to stagger their meal breaks, and have concluded them by 9.00 p.m.

One pair had taken a two-hour break, well exceeding the official allowance of a maximum of sixty minutes, between approximately 7.30 p.m. and 9.30 p.m. They'd made a ten-mile round trip to buy kebabs. At 8.58 p.m., the other pair, both PCSOs, took a ninety-minute break that overlapped with their colleagues. At least one officer should have been on duty in the City Room – one of the busiest exit routes – from 10.00 p.m., as people started to leave the concert, but there were no BTP staff at all present.

Gradually, the room began to fill up with parents collecting their children from the concert. At 10.15 p.m. one couple arrived and headed up onto the mezzanine level to wait. When they passed Abedi who was sitting, alone, near a wall, the astute woman asked her partner why he thought Abedi was at a 'children's concert' with a giant rucksack. Why indeed. Clearly concerned, the brave, conscientious man approached Abedi and challenged him. He asked what was in his rucksack. Abedi didn't answer or make eye contact. The man tackled him again: 'It doesn't look very good, you know, what you see with bombs and such… you, with a rucksack like this in a place like this. What are you doing?' This time, Abedi answered. He said he was waiting for someone. Then he asked what the time was. The man said he didn't know.

Troubled, the man walked away and looked around for a police officer to approach. There wasn't one. Instead, he spoke to the security officer, who said he was already aware of Abedi. The whistleblower told the inquiry that the security guard didn't seem interested or share his concerns. He felt 'fobbed off'. The security guard has denied this, insisting he'd reassured the man that he would report Abedi. He said he told him not to worry as he did not to want him to be concerned and worry other people.

Granted, he did try to get the attention of his boss, thirty metres away, by raising his hand. The boss did not see. The guard didn't have a radio and he didn't think he could leave his post. Eight minutes later, he alerted a radio-carrying colleague. By now, Abedi was sitting on the steps leading down to the city hall from the mezzanine. He appeared sweaty and fidgety. The second security guard admitted to the inquiry that he had a 'bad feeling' about Abedi. But he was wary of being labelled racist if he made the wrong call. CCTV images had shown the two guards talking, glancing across at Abedi. This second security guard tried, several times, to get through to the control room on his radio but was unable to make contact. He then, it seems, gave up trying.

CCTV footage shows the second guard walking away from the City Room. Those two security guards, with so much responsibility, were just eighteen and nineteen.

At 10.30 p.m. Abedi rose to his feet. He walked down the stairs and across the City Room towards the Arena entrance. According to witnesses, he was on his phone. He was smiling. He stood, motionless, in the middle of the room surrounded by innocent kids, teens and doting parents and blew himself up.

At the sound of the explosion, the four BTP officers – who had been standing together at Victoria Station – ran to the City Room to help victims. Yes, they were first on the scene. Yes, they administered first aid. Afterwards, some of them accepted accolades and awards and were hailed as heroes. But had they been there earlier, on duty, as instructed, could they have thwarted Abedi's murderous mission?

Surely, the true heroes were those who tried to raise the alarm about Abedi and others, like Robert Grew, who ran towards the atrocity. But their bravery, their foresight, has never been officially recognised.

Countless other errors were also uncovered: the security perimeter for bag searches didn't stretch as far as the outlying areas of the arena. That's how Abedi could enter the City Room without having his bag searched. There was also little communication or cooperation between the three organisations responsible for running the event that night; SMG (the owner and operator of the arena); Showsec (the company contracted for crowd management and security) and British Transport Police. Unlicensed staff were both carrying out bag checks and monitoring CCTV monitoring without having undergone training.

Sir John said, 'I am satisfied that there were a number of missed opportunities to alter the course of what happened that night. More should have been done.' The most striking of those missed opportunities and the one that was likely to have made a significant difference, he said, was the attempt by the parent to raise concerns. He 'formed the view that Abedi might "let a bomb off". That was sadly all too prescient and makes all the more distressing the fact that no effective steps were taken as a result of the efforts made.' Sir John said 'disruptive intervention' should have been taken against Abedi and lives could have been saved as a result. It's likely that the terrorist would still have detonated his device, he said, but the loss of life and injury was highly likely to have been less. I realise it's something we'll never know.

Sir John pointed out that regulations for issues like food hygiene were rigorous. 'I do not see why prevention of terrorist attacks should not be treated in the same way,' he concluded.

Quite. Security arrangements for the Arena, he said, 'should have prevented or minimised the devastating impact of the attack. They failed to do so.' I was impressed. Sir John did not attempt to sugarcoat his findings or spare anyone's feelings. As bad as the night had been, these facts and findings needed to be heard. As Sir John himself said, it wasn't about finger-pointing.

Journalists asked me for my reaction. I said, 'I want them to apologise, learn from events and put plans in place to ensure that nothing like this ever happens again.' I felt weary and exhausted.

But I'd long realised that getting angry and allowing bitterness to take hold wouldn't do any good. I'd acknowledge these thoughts and feelings as they occurred to me, then let them go. What's done is done. You can't change the past. You can, however, change the future. I fully support Figen Murray – the mother of Martyn Hett, aged twenty-nine, who died on the night – who has been campaigning tirelessly for Martyn's Law or a Protect Duty. This new legislation would ensure all public venues had appropriate security procedures in place.

A month later, I wheeled myself into the inquiry and took the stand. I described how it had felt at the moment of detonation – like being hit by a ten-ton truck. How I knew I was losing a lot of blood. How I knew both I, and Eve, were dying. I revealed that Eve had been covered up twice. 'People were looking at her injury and saying that it was not survivable. They just covered her up even though she was alive and they weren't qualified to make that kind of choice. Even if they were, you do your damnedest to ensure survivability and preservation of life. You don't make that decision yourself and walk away. I don't think I will ever get my head around that.' I recalled the utter despair I felt for myself and my daughter. 'To go through that, to know that you're dying and to be left alone and to know that nobody's coming... it's an awful thing to go through.'

And my comment that it was adding 'insult to our injury' for the families of the deceased and survivors that medals had been given to 'certain professionals where the evidence shows their professional and moral duty was not acted upon appropriately' was widely reported in the media.

Sir John established the timings of how the night unfolded. The bomb had gone off at 10.31 p.m. But I hadn't arrived at the clearing station until 11.25 p.m., almost a full hour later. I left for hospital at 12.24 a.m., arriving at 12.32 a.m. – two hours and one minute after the bombing.

Afterwards, I wheeled myself out. It was done. All I could do now was wait for the reports to come out.

I turned my attentions back to Kilimanjaro. Two more practice expeditions were planned – a five-day trek along the West Highland Way in Scotland in early October 2021 and a climb up Snowdon the following March. We were all set for Scotland when I fell ill.

Yes, sepsis had got me – for the fifth time. While the others set off, with SIA ambassador and Paralympian Karen Darke taking my place in the wheelchair to allow the team to practise, I was at Salford Royal being pumped full of lifesaving antibiotics. This time, I'm pleased to say my treatment was second to none. But I could see the concern on Gabby's face. If this happened halfway up Kilimanjaro it was game over. 'I'll be fine,' I insisted. And I really meant it.

Just weeks later, 'Martin's Mountain Afternoon Tea' reception was held in London with the entire team, sponsors and partners. Andy was round at Mum's that night and thought she was going to burst when I appeared on television on the same table as our royal patron, Anne, Princess Royal.

On the Monday morning, I made another appearance on *BBC Breakfast* to promote the event. I was delighted when the BBC announced they'd like to cover the trip and make a documentary about it.

Gabby whisked us away to the Lake District so I could rest before training restarted. Mum texted to ask what the cottage was like.

'Have a lovely few days,' she'd said. 'I'll see you when you're back.' Her health hadn't been great lately. I don't think she'd ever got over the shock of her son and granddaughter being so badly injured.

Until the attack, Eve and I had stayed at Mum's every single weekend. She'd loved having the company. By then she was crippled with arthritis and struggling to walk. While visiting me in hospital, she needed a wheelchair to get around. After a double knee replacement in 2018, Mum was desperate to retire and she moved to a smaller terraced house to be mortgage-free. We were all concerned about the steep stairs but she insisted she'd be fine. Like many people, covid had hit her hard. She missed all her old neighbours.

In September, we'd gone out to celebrate her seventieth birthday. We noticed that just walking from the car to the restaurant entrance she was breathless and had to sit down to rest. I remember seeing the concern on Gabby's face as she helped her. 'Are you often like this, Janice?' she'd asked gently.

Mum shook her head. 'I'm fine,' she insisted. It's clear now she wasn't being honest. But that's Mum. Stoic and stubborn (and people wonder where I get it from…).

On the second evening of our mini-break, Andy rang. 'Is Mum with you?' he asked.

'Andy, I'm in the Lakes,' I said. 'Why would Mum be with me?'

'Right, we've got an issue,' he said. I could hear the concern in his voice. He and Danny were outside Mum's. The house was in darkness. Mum hadn't been on WhatsApp for twenty-four hours. 'We think she might have fallen,' he said.

My scalp prickled. 'I'll stay on the line while you go in,' I said. *Please have dozed off. Please be at a friend's house. Please be OK, Mum.* The kitchen was empty. Andy went into the lounge and put the light on. Mum was on the couch. I waited to hear her cry out in surprise. To exclaim they'd frightened the life out of her sneaking in like that. But there was nothing.

My lovely, amazing, devoted Mum had died in her sleep, watching TV. The remote control was on her knee. A post-mortem revealed cor pulmonale – or pulmonary heart disease, also known as right-sided heart failure. Doctors assured us her passing would have been calm and peaceful. It was how you'd want to go if your time was up – but it was just so sudden. There was no warning. No chance to tell her how much she meant to me. How much I loved her. No goodbye.

Oh, Mum.

I've heard people talk about grief causing a physical pain in the heart. But I'd never understood it. Until now. There were times the crushing sensation in my chest literally took my breath away.

In a daze of grief, we planned her funeral. I was adamant about one thing. I was going to join my brothers in carrying her coffin. I could see confusion pass over the undertaker's face. 'Erm, this isn't something we've been asked to do before,' he began. 'I'm not sure…'

I put my hand up. 'It was done for Prince Philip's funeral. They carried the coffin at waist height. If it can be done for Prince Philip, it can be done for me mum.'

And, so, with a bit of help from my friends, all three Hibbert boys carried Mum's coffin into the crematorium to the sounds of 'Go Your Own Way', by Fleetwood Mac – one of her favourite songs. Danny was at the front with the undertaker, with Andy and me at the rear. Andy carried his corner at waist height. I had my corner wedged onto my shoulder and held it with both hands.

My friend Mark, one of the Kilimanjaro team, held onto the front of my wheelchair to ensure it didn't tip up backwards with the extra weight, while Steve pushed me. Progress was slow but we did it.

The service was a celebration of her life. We chose a lovely photo of her from her sixtieth birthday for the order of service. I remembered the day so well. We'd taken her to Bettys for a birthday tea. Eve, then eight, had been there too, of course. Such special times.

We knew Mum wouldn't want maudlin, weepy songs, so we chose 'Red Light Spells Danger' by Billy Ocean and Take That's version of 'Could It Be Magic'. As the curtains closed, I bowed my head and cried.

I have a little shrine at home. It includes an urn with some of her ashes, all the Mother's Day cards she treasured over the years and my favourite photos of her. While clearing her house we found our locks of baby hair: 'She was so proud of you all,' her friends told us after the service. I miss her so much. Always will.

I knew that one of the hardest things about Kilimanjaro would be doing it without Mum in my life. When I was in Australia, I'd been facetiming her endlessly, sending countless videos of me performing miracles. She told me she'd cried watching me standing for the first time. But even though she'd gone, when we did the Snowdon training, I felt her presence once again.

The trip came in March 2022, shortly after I was delighted to be appointed vice president of the SIA. Everything went like clockwork. The weather was beautiful and I was surrounded by all these wonderful people who had given up their time and weekends to support me. As the sun split through the clouds, I heard her voice, as clear as anything, say, 'I'm really proud of you.' I stopped dead in my tracks. Then broke down, sobbing. She was still with me.

Exhausted, but triumphant at how well we had done, we finally made it back to our cars. As the team dispersed, we said our goodbyes to Caroline and Stuart. I was about to transfer into my car when I shifted in my seat. Something didn't feel right. Twisting, I peered down my back. *Oh, bloody hell.* My bowels had emptied. It was like the journey back from Australia – 'Nightmare on the plane – part two'. *What do I do? What do I do?* Chris had suggested we try out the new bowel management method that morning in my tent before setting off. However, at the time, nothing had happened. We had waited a minute, then tried again. 'Maybe my bowel isn't ready to empty?' I suggested. Time was ticking so we decided to crack on. I learned afterwards that my bowel, unused to the method, had been refusing to play ball that morning. However, the physical exertion of climbing up and down Snowdon had got things moving, shall we say.

'What are you going to do?' asked Steve.

I looked around, desperately. 'There's not a lot I can do, is there?' I cried. 'I'm in the middle of a bloody car park.' Then, call it telepathy, Caroline and Stuart's car slowed, turned around, and drove back.

'Everything OK, Martin?' Stuart called.

I gave them an unconvincing thumbs up. In a flash they were over. 'I've had an explosion,' I confessed, 'but it's fine. I'll sort it when I'm home.'

They immediately fired into action mode. 'Right, in the back,' they said, manoeuvring me into the boot of my Range Rover. They clambered in and closed the door. Then with a snapping of rubber gloves, it was all systems go. Expertly and briskly, they stripped me off, cleaned me up and rolled me this way and that, before re-dressing me in fresh clothing.

Steve had to stand outside, trying to look inconspicuous, as the car rocked from side to side with all the movement inside. Thank God for blacked-out windows. Finally, the door opened and we emerged, red-faced and sweaty. Heaven only knows what people thought we were up to in there. I drove home as fresh as a daisy and counting my blessings. I bought Caroline flowers to say thank-you – even though she playfully hit me with them and insisted I was being ridiculous. They really were true friends.

As the departure date grew closer, we stepped up the publicity efforts. I appeared on countless breakfast TV shows, speaking ever more passionately about the reasons for this bonkers idea. 'I'm lucky. It's a miracle I survived and I've had love, care and support to get me to this point. But during my recovery, I was shocked to learn that 2,500 people suffer a spinal cord injury in the UK each year. Yet only one in three receive treatment at a specialist spinal injury centre. What about those living on the thirtieth floor of a council block with a broken lift? Or those left lying in their own mess for two days because carers have covid? That's what this is about. When it comes to life after injury, I want everyone to have hope for a better tomorrow.

'Yes,' I admitted, getting into my stride. 'I'm hoping that being on that summit, looking down on the world, will help me put to bed a lot of the horrors of what happened that night. But this isn't just about me climbing a mountain. It's about me saying to other people living with a disability, "Look what you can do with the right team and support around you." And it's also saying to the government, "If you invest in everybody who is disabled – not just the one in three – look at what can happen. You can do the impossible." We'll have more people back working, paying taxes, growing the economy, as opposed to taking up hospital beds or surviving on benefits.'

I felt like Winston Churchill making one of his famous war speeches. 'Dream, believe, achieve,' became my mantra. 'If you can dream it, you can do it. Anything is possible.'

On one show, I received a montage of good luck messages from Manchester United players thanking me for my incredible support over the years and now saying it was their turn to support me. There were also good-luck messages from actor and adventurer Brian Blessed, wheelchair basketball player and TV presenter Ade Adepitan and explorer and presenter Ben Fogle, whose message was, 'You're my hero. Everything about this extraordinary story is as inspiring as it is humbling.' I nearly crashed the car when Zoe Ball issued a good luck message on her BBC Radio 2 breakfast show.

We were flying out on 2 June and would have two days to prepare before the hard work began. Laying out my mounds of kit, clothes and essentials, I couldn't believe this was finally happening. Once again, I felt a pang that Mum wouldn't be there to see me do this. 'She'd have been so proud,' my brothers said. Remembering her ashes, I had a brainwave. Now, Mum hated the cold and would kill me if I distributed all of her ashes on the summit. But I could scatter *some*. I went online and ordered a scatter tube. I lovingly packed the precious cargo in my hand luggage.

I smiled at her photo. 'You ready, Mum?' She was going to be with me after all.

17

On Top of the World

In one of my favourite photos from the Tanzanian trip I'm sitting bolt upright in my wheelchair, gazing at a snow-capped Kilimanjaro rising majestically on the horizon.

It was the first day of our arrival following the flight to Kilimanjaro airport and transfer to the lodge at Moshi. We'd had a busy few hours unpacking, sorting kit and – the most important job – assembling and checking my precious trike. After briefings with the expedition leader, we'd assembled for group photos taken against the amazing backdrop. As everyone dispersed for dinner, I'd hung behind, turned my wheelchair back and continued to look.

It was an incredible sight, dominating the landscape. And it was even more amazing to think it was formed a million years ago as a result of volcanic activity. I was also giving this miracle of Mother Nature a right good talking-to. 'OK, I'm here,' I began, in a low voice, so no one would overhear. 'I've done it. I've put all the training in. I've given you respect. You need to give me respect now.' I remembered everything Karl had warned about. The thin air, the burning muscles, the exhaustion, the constant swirling of emotions. 'I don't care what you throw at me. I'm going to do it. I'm trained. I'm ready for this.'

I closed my eyes, sensing Mum and Grandad. I felt the good-luck hugs from Eve, Gabby, Karl, my brothers. I recalled all the wonderful messages that were still flowing in, from people with SCIs to celebrities. And I thought of the countless people who would, hopefully, be helped by fundraising. There were those already in wheelchairs and spinal injury units, as well as the others who weren't there yet but would be, one day. I'd been one of the latter group until 10.31 p.m. on 22 May 2017. Blissfully living my able-bodied life, walking, running, weeing, pooing. Never dreaming it would, in an instant, be taken away from me. No one ever does. In that moment, I vowed that nothing would stop me and Mum reaching the top. 'I'm going to kick your ass,' I promised. Behind me, Graeme had turned to see where I was and taken the snap without me realising. I treasure the image.

My back was broad from all the training. I was sitting tall, shoulders back. Ready and waiting to take on this immense challenge we'd spent two years preparing for. Since returning from Tanzania I've faced countless nerve-wracking moments – making presentations to thousands of people, meeting government ministers in the Houses of Parliament. If I need motivation, I always take a deep breath and conjure that image. How strong I felt in that moment. I'd never been more ready in my life.

Let's do this.

The BBC did countless interviews for their documentary *Martin's Mountain: Climbing Kilimanjaro*. In the footage of me speaking to camera, strength and determination ooze out of every pore. 'I survived for this moment – to show how we can celebrate and embrace disability. Look at what we can do with the right support. We can literally climb mountains. I'm ready to smash it now.'

Not everyone had the same belief in their abilities. Each week in the altitude chamber, remember, at least one of the team had struggled and been asked to step outside so their oxygen levels could recover. The scientists had explained this had nothing to do with levels of fitness or ability. Our physiologies are all unique and we all react to new environments in different ways. Steve, one of the fittest people I know, was particularly vulnerable. 'I'd found the altitude training hard,' he recalls. 'Afterwards, I'd develop a proper, raging headache that completely debilitated me. The only time I didn't was when I was pushing myself exceptionally hard. However, I knew that the climb had to be done at a very slow pace to allow us to acclimatise. So, I think, deep down I always had that fear.'

It took a four-hour drive to reach Rongai Gate, where our squad of guides and porters was waiting. They thronged around. You could feel the joy, the overwhelming excitement in the air. They had done this climb countless times, but they were brimming over with bonhomie, zest and enthusiasm.

'Martin's!' someone called.

'Mountain!' they responded, as one, before breaking into a lively song and dance. Grinning, we all clapped along. It was like being at the best party ever. And if they were like this at the start, how on earth would they be at the summit?

The organisation was slick and well-practised. Each day, the porters would pack up the tents and stride on ahead, ready to set up the next camp further along the trek. But it was important for us, the climbers, to ascend slowly. 'Pole, pole,' (pronounced 'Po-lay') they'd call to each other in Swahili. 'Slowly, slowly.' The speed never changed. They knew exactly what they were doing. Slow and steady. I pumped the handles of the tricycle. The wheels effortlessly glided over boulders. My love for cars now extended to chairs and trikes. Amazing piece of engineering, I'd find myself thinking.

We stopped regularly to gather everyone and swig water. Staying hydrated was crucial in staving off both exhaustion and altitude wobbles. At every break, Chris would check in, unzipping the leg of my salopettes to place his hand on my shin and calf. Then he'd slip his hand under my top layers to compare the temperature. 'All good,' he'd say, reassuringly. If I was too cold, I'd need warming up urgently. Too hot, we'd need to strip off my upper layers.

We'd also do a virtual top-to-toe scan. How was I feeling? Comfortable? Any itching? Chafing? He'd check my catheter bag. 'Good, good,' he'd murmur, reassuringly.

At camp that night I was staggered at the quality of the food. I'd honestly envisaged surviving on spatchcock rat and rice. But the meals included delicious pizzas and chicken and chips. 'How can you cook this on a mountain?' I gasped. It was a question that was never answered. They literally cooked in the ground. It was like magic.

Turning in that night, I felt a surge of gratitude for Chris curled up in my tent. My SCI-friendly camp bed took up so much room that Chris was in the porch section. He was an outdoor soul and didn't feel the cold, he assured me. "Night Chris – and thank you,' I'd said, as he turned our flashlamp out.

"Night Martin. And no worries,' he replied.

Elsewhere, Steve was already in trouble. 'By the end of the first day, I had the worst headache ever,' he remembers. He quietly confided in the medics who gave him medication and urged him to lie down in his tent in the hope his body would acclimatise. Sure enough, by 4.00 a.m., the headache had eased. As dawn broke, he felt great, at least for a while.

Every morning, the crew drawn from the local people would gather for a team song and dance. The sheer va-va-voom of each and every person was infectious. They had very little in the way of money or possessions but they were living their best life. We'd all join in – clapping, dancing and punching the air. Apart from poor Chris, that is. Having got me toileted, dressed and ready to face the day, he then had to sort himself.

The weather turned wet, grey and misty and there was a communal rustle as waterproofs were retrieved from rucksacks. I was insulated to within an inch of my life. On top of all my layers I wore a waterproof poncho. Not one drop of rain penetrated my armour. I pumped the handles confidently and happily as we moved further through the forests.

Behind me, Steve was struggling. The others noticed he'd gone quiet. 'As soon as we started climbing again, the headache returned,' he says. 'It felt like my head was in a vice and each step I took turned it tighter and tighter. The medics suggested taking it slowly and seeing if things settled once I'd reached second camp and had a chance to lie down. But by the time we got there I thought my head was going to explode. The guides did some cognitive tests – asked me to walk in a straight line, follow their finger with my eyes as they moved it from side to side.'

Steve thought he'd aced the tests. The two medics exchanged words. Then they turned to him. 'Off. Now.'

He'd wanted to do this both for me and as a tribute to his late wife. I knew it would hit him hard. I'd never seen him so dejected and miserable. 'I'm so sorry, Martin,' he said, hugging me. 'I've let you down.'

I hugged him even tighter. 'Mate, you've been by my side every step of the way,' I said into his chest. 'I couldn't have done it without you.' This moment, like every minute of our trip, was being caught on film. Most of the time, I hardly noticed the film crew, but now I did. 'I'm gutted for him,' I said. Then my composure cracked. 'Give me two minutes,' I said. On film, as Steve is led down the mountain, you can clearly hear me crying loudly in my tent. For those few moments, I was engulfed in sheer and utter terror. Would I succumb too and have to pull out? Would all this time, effort and money have been for nothing? I took a deep breath. Get a grip, Martin, I told myself. You haven't got the time or energy for a panic attack.

I remembered the vow I'd made to the mountain. I closed my eyes and thought of Mum. Eve. Gabby, Grandad, Alfie. I imagined them all saying the same thing. 'You've got this, Martin. You've got this.'

The mood was subdued in camp that night. Everyone was thinking the same thing. Bloody hell. If it's got Steve – Mr Fitness himself – on day two, what chance have the rest of us got? The miserable weather hadn't helped. We'd arrived at camp to find our tent had leaked like a sieve. I say 'our' tent. My bit was as dry as a bone. Chris's sleeping quarters were three inches deep in water. He spent ages wringing out sodden kit. The team strapped a groundsheet over the tent to prevent any more water coming in but Chris had to set up his damp bed elsewhere. I learned afterwards he already hadn't been sleeping well – which is another symptom of being at altitude – and he'd woken some mornings feeling nauseous. The medics assured him it was a low level risk but they'd keep monitoring him.

As we progressed, the landscape continually changed. Dense rainforests made way for moorlands, farmlands, rocky paths. With every metre we climbed the vegetation and oxygen became sparser. Communication with home wasn't great but the team leaders were managing to keep our loved ones updated with brief messages. Gabby was keeping everyone on the WhatsApp group and Twitter feed updated. I had no idea that thousands of people were following our every move.

By camp four, we really did feel we were on a mountain. A lunar landscape spread out before us. You could see the snow line up ahead. And above that, the route to the summit. This was going to be the hardest part. Up ahead were the 'switchbacks' that Karl had warned me about. Huge expanses of slippery shale. Imagine a volcanic beach in the Canary Islands. Now tip it on its side and try to walk up it.

We all gathered in the mess tent for dinner and a final team briefing from Kat – at this stage it was too cold to be out in the open. We'd need an early night. Tomorrow, before sunrise, we'd be ascending. The group leader had decided that, because we were going at different paces, we'd go in two groups. The first group would start at 3 a.m. Then the guides, with me in my wheelchair, would follow an hour later. We needed to go at our own pace, ask for help if we needed it. If we got a tap on the shoulder from the guides we were to go straight back down. We exchanged glances.

Imagine coming so close to the summit and not being able to make it.

Chris was about to find out. Within minutes, he went from well to unwell. 'Suddenly, it was as if someone had put a vice around my head,' he recalls now. 'There was the most terrible build-up of pressure. My vision started to close in and I was staggering like a drunk man.' The medics made the call. Chris couldn't continue. Our brief, hurried, goodbye is heartbreaking. The film shows a tearful Chris crawl into my tent for a hug. You see my hands reach out. Then I'm not just crying but proper bawling. Great big heaving, shuddering, sobs. That was my lowest point. I'd lost my best friend and my nurse.

Alone in my tent that night, I felt consumed by utter terror. Everyone was sleeping, garnering their energy for the big push the following morning. For the first time in my life, I felt scared of the dark. I kept a light on. I was alone in a tent, high up a mountain, in the middle of a strange continent. Outside, it was pitch black and freezing. I'd never felt so alone. From deep within, I felt a familiar stirring. '*You idiot,*' Bad/Sad Martin jeered. '*What were you thinking? Did you honestly think you'd...*'

Grabbing my phone, I jabbed at the screen. I'd downloaded some treasures before leaving the UK just in case there were moments like this. Press. Press. Press.

...Making a fool of yourself and everyone else...

And suddenly, there it was. The opening chords of the *Fawlty Towers* theme – a famous sitcom from the eighties. I focused on the screen. On Basil Fawlty. On Sybil. They drowned out Bad/Sad Martin's taunts. I couldn't make out what he was saying any more. Within a few minutes, he'd settled down. After *Fawlty Towers* I watched *Laurel and Hardy*. My mouth twitched. I smiled. I even chuckled. I imagined I was back on the couch with Grandad Bill. On my other side was Grandad Bob, urging me not to wait for my ship to come in. And up there, on the summit, waiting for me, was Mum. By the time the camp stirred into life, I hadn't slept a wink but felt invigorated. They say laughter is the best medicine and they're absolutely right.

Stuart stepped in to help me get dressed and empty my catheter. Before succumbing to altitude sickness, Chris, bless him, had sorted my bowels and my kit, laying out everything I would need. Because, at this height, even just dressing was an ordeal. Even just dressing was an ordeal. The slightest movement left you out of breath. It was like starring in your own slow-motion movie. Finally, I was in my wheelchair with my team of guides around me. We all switched our headlamps on. 'Let's do this,' I said.

Gradually, the light changed. TV presenter Dan Walker, who had done the climb previously, had told me, 'Martin, make sure you look up and see the sun rising. It's the most beautiful thing you will ever see.' And he was right. We paused for a few moments so I could take in the breathtaking view and capture it on my phone. Then we pressed on.

Wispy, gossamer clouds floated around our heads, as we focused on trying to ascend the steepest, slipperiest slope imaginable. It was like trying to wheel myself through thick, treacly gravel. My arms were pumping like pistons. Back and forth. Back and forth. But my wheels, like everyone else's feet, were sinking helplessly. We were taking one step forward, then slithering back three. It was exhausting. Relentless. Soul-destroying.

'How much further?' I gasped at one point. The lead guide smiled. 'Twenty minutes,' he assured me. I got my head down. Half an hour later, I asked again. 'Twenty minutes,' he repeated. When he gave the same answer an hour later, I could feel my patience wearing thin. 'You said that last time,' I cried indignantly. I sounded like a petulant child. Progress was painfully slow. 'Pole, pole,' they said. 'Pole, pole...'

But the clock was ticking. If we didn't reach the summit by 12.30 p.m. it was game over. There wouldn't be time to safely descend back down to camp. At one point I couldn't help it. 'We're not going to make it, are we?' I asked, dreading his answer.

But the lead porter responded with a determined, 'Yes, we are. Just twenty more minutes.'

I could hear Mum in my head urging me on, encouraging me. 'Come on, son, you're so close. Almost there. Almost there...'

Finally, finally, we'd cleared the switchbacks and hit the rocks and boulders. Together, the team dug in, lifted me, pulled me, heaved me over treacherous boulders and crevices. Watching the film now, it looks precarious. But I never once felt in danger. Just ahead was the sign for the summit, Gilman's Point. I was pumping the push-pull levers so furiously I wouldn't have been surprised to see them snap off in my hands. The porters in front pulled. From behind, they pushed. With a satisfying bump, my front wheel rose and cleared the final ridge. My back wheels followed. And bloody hell, we'd done it. The team jumped up and down punching the air. I lifted my arms, exhausted.

Top of the world. I really was on top of the world. I rummaged in my bag for my phone and my precious travel urn of mum's ashes then turned to the BBC camera.

'We've done it. We're at the top of Kilimanjaro.' My voice sounds thin and weak. I'm out of breath just speaking. The air is thick with cloud. 'Sadly, my mum passed away in November. She was immensely proud. I said she was going to be with me and she is. I said when we got to the top I'd spread some ashes, play our favourite tune, so I'm going to do that now.'

Shakily, I fumble on my phone. The strains of The Carpenters' 'For All We Know' float through the air. 'This is for you, Mum,' I say. I'm so weak I can hardly prise the lid from the tube. But finally, with a soft pop, it's free. I raise it, tilt it then, with a huge effort, scatter the precious contents. 'Love you, Mum,' I say quietly, sniffing and wiping my tear-stained cheeks with gloved hands.

We grabbed some more photos: a picture of me giving a thumbs-up to the camera (the photo which appears on the cover of this book) and another of me proudly holding my United flag aloft. But I could sense the porters starting to shuffle. 'I'm fine, honestly,' I insisted. I felt so great that I was tempted to join the others at the other summit point (there are three altogether) a little further along. As I watched I could see a bit of commotion. *What the heck's going on up there?* From where I was sitting, it looked like Caroline was struggling to walk and two other members of the crew were having to carry Rob. I watched, bewildered.

Caroline had experienced a dramatic onset of peripheral oedema – fluid build-up in her lower legs. 'I felt like the Michelin man – like my trousers were going to burst,' she recalls. Mark's face was swelling up. And, terrifyingly, Rob suffered swelling of the brain – cerebral oedema – causing him to vomit dramatically over the side of a cliff and had to be carried down to camp.

Chris laughs now: 'We were going down like flies. But the one person who didn't suffer any adverse effects was you, Martin. The one we'd all been worried about.' Poor Chris. The medics and porters had all been so surprised he didn't make it. As a sole climber, he'd have completed it no problem. But he'd sacrificed himself to get me up there. 'It was a real kick,' he admits. 'But, from the beginning, my job was always just to get you to the top. I was your stepping stone.'

I'll for ever be grateful to him – and my entire team. They did everything in their power to get me up there. The last five years had led to this moment. A part of Mum's spirit and my own heart will always remain up there.

I barely remember the descent. By this point, there was nothing left in the tank. Struggling to sit up, I was wobbling dangerously. Caroline and Stuart exchanged concerned glances. They admit now they were all worried sick that I was going to fall at the final hurdle. 'You'd used everything you had to get to that summit,' Stuart says. 'The last time I'd seen you so weak and helpless was when you first arrived on my ward. I was terrified that you'd come down with an infection or skin breakdown.' Back at camp they checked my skin, emptied my catheter bag and tucked me into bed. I briefly rang Gabby on a satellite phone and triumphantly gasped,

'I've done it.' (She said I sounded both breathless and drunk.) Then I slept like a baby.

Meanwhile, back at the hotel, Chris and Steve were waiting anxiously for news. With no communication they had no way of knowing if we'd made it. So, the look on their faces when we finally returned, exhausted but triumphant, will stay with me for ever – as will the friendships carved on that trip. As Chris said in the documentary, 'Friends forged under pressure always last.' We've become a brotherhood for life.

And for those who'd seen me at my lowest, the trip also provided a sense of closure and hope. Caroline says now, 'I could never not have done this trip with you. It was a great way to cement our journey and our friendship. I was the first person to teach you how to sit on the edge of a bed and transfer from bed to wheelchair. I was also that person who then got to the top of Kilimanjaro with you. There are not many people who will see that kind of recovery with their patients. So, yes, it was an absolute honour to be there.'

I predicted we'd return home different people and we did. Climbing Kilimanjaro opened up our horizons. We met the most wonderful people who had nothing in the way of material possessions. But they had happiness in abundance. Yes, reaching that summit was the whole purpose of our trip. But our eyes had been opened in so many ways. I returned home, more convinced than ever, that life was precious. A gift to be treasured.

I was stunned to learn that Manchester poet Tony Walsh had written a poem to commemorate my trip. The BBC used it to close the documentary. Over dramatic footage of the climb and the most beautiful inspiring music, Tony narrated the words in his own inimitable, passionate, Mancunian way. I can think of no better way to finish this chapter.

Everyday Mountains

From a single act of violence, and the 22 we lost
The hundreds, maybe thousands, who still pay a daily cost

There comes choirs, there comes music, there comes
  campaigns, there comes stories
There comes glades of light and daily fights, and love in all
  its glory

There comes Martin, in his wheelchair, with just one thing
  on his mind
And "Dream! Believe! Achieve!" he says, and "Onwards!
  Forwards! Climb!"
And with northern bloody-mindedness, "As crazy as this
  sounds
We'll raise hope, we'll raise awareness. We will raise a
  million pounds!"
Those who saw him at his lowest, at the very gates of hell
Those who stitched him back together said, "You're mad!'
  'We'll climb as well!"

From a basecamp on a bombsite, this is wheelchair v volcano
Yes, it's rough and yes it's tough, but Martin's often heard to
  say though:
"Climb for dignity, humanity, and all like me who say:
Believe in us achieving. We climb mountains everyday!"

Over rock and over rivers, and through heat and sheeting
  rain
Through blood and sweat and fears, and through sickness
  and through pain
Over boulders, aching shoulders, something holds us,
  through the snow
Something in us, deep within us. We dig in and on we go.

And he made it! To the summit! And united with his Mum
And he raised a flag to Manchester with "Look mum, what
  I've done!"

And to those who would divide us and spread hatred all
  around
This says "Love can conquer mountains, and it's never
  coming down!"
And it's strong and it can catch us, it can lift us to the top
And Martin? He's just starting and he's never gonna stop!

From a single act of violence, comes a simple act of love
We rise, we rise, we rise, we rise, we rise. We rise above.

18

I'm Vindicated... and Trolled

We flew home to a heroes' welcome.

Summit pictures and video footage of me had appeared all over national newspapers, news bulletins, websites and social media pages while we were still on the journey home. Donations surged but there was still a long way to go.

The following morning, I was on the *BBC Breakfast* sofa. I laughed when presenters, John Kay and Sally Nugent, asked if I was tired. 'If my body had an orange light it would be flashing a 'fuel low' warning!' I replied. The early interview was worth it to keep spreading the word and encourage more donations. 'The hard work starts now,' I vowed. 'We've climbed a mountain – now we have to *move* mountains to get the changes we need.'

As well as donations and sponsorship, we'd also been encouraging people to take part in the #MY19 challenge – doing everything from running nineteen miles to baking nineteen cakes to tie in with the 19,000 feet height of Kilimanjaro. Chris's son, Cian, aged just six, climbed the equivalent of 19,000 feet on mountains in Britain and Ireland – including Snowdon. My amazing team at Hudgell Solicitors, now representing me, along with other survivors and families, raised a staggering £100,000 through various challenges.

Chris himself signed up for new challenges to make up for not reaching the summit. He and Graeme completed a fifty-kilometre ultra-marathon together and the following summer, he completed a double marathon. He dreams of returning to Kilimanjaro and I have no doubt that without me to look after he'll make it to the top.

The money raised went through the half a million pounds mark, then the three quarters of a million pounds. We were well on our way. As Stuart says, 'Martin's Mountain was a true example of how terrorism doesn't divide people, it actually brings them together.'

That closeness and positivity helped me cope with the knowledge that the publication of the second and third reports into the Inquiry were imminent.

For the past four years, I'd been vilified on social media for my regular outbursts about how victims and survivors had been let down that night. My comment about the emergency services having blood on their hands had led to a lot of criticism. Both the public and workers in public services would message, 'How dare you? These people saved your life.' I needed to stay busy. Occupied. I threw myself into visiting Eve and delivering motivational talks.

In November 2022, the waiting ended with the publication of the second report. I braced myself to hear Sir John's opening remarks on the news. He said, 'I saw CCTV evidence and video from body-worn cameras at the City Room that showed clearly the appalling aftermath of the explosion. It showed those who had died within seconds of the explosion. It showed victims with appalling injuries.' Me and Eve... 'Those who have listened to the evidence will not be surprised that I am highly critical of many aspects of the rescue operation. While some of the decisions made by some commanders were overly cautious, individual firefighters and paramedics were ready and willing to carry out their job of protecting and saving life. There were significant failings by a number of organisations in preparation and training for an emergency such as this, and in their actions on the night of the attack ... Some may think that to criticise individuals who were faced with an extremely difficult situation is harsh, but we rely on people in command positions to make the right decisions when faced with a complex emergency.'

In the report, he explained that the Joint Emergency Services Interoperability Principles (JESIP), introduced after the 7/7 London terror attack, failed 'almost completely'. He continued, 'JESIP is designed to ensure that any rescue attempt involving more than one of the emergency services is coordinated so they all follow the same plan and share information so that well-informed decisions can be taken. Had JESIP worked, things could have been very different.' There would have been a joint assessment of risk taken by all the emergency services. There would have been more paramedics in the City Room using their skills to triage and, where necessary, using their life-saving skills to assist those who couldn't wait to be removed from the City Room before they received treatment. Fire-fighters would have arrived on the scene to use their considerable skills to ensure an organised and safe removal of the injured to the station entrance where they could receive assessment and treatment pending a rapid transfer to hospital.

That's what should have happened.

'Instead, we heard heartbreaking evidence of the injured and the rescuers who were in the City Room hearing the sirens of ambulances, knowing paramedics were close by, expecting their imminent arrival, only for them not to arrive in the sort of numbers which were needed. Had fire fighters got to the City Room as soon as they could have done, they would have removed the injured using proper equipment which would have been safe and quick. Instead, the injured had to be removed on railings and pieces of cardboard which were uncomfortable and unsafe. Painfully – and inevitably – this meant that it took longer for each patient to be removed.'

And there, in those words, we had it. Vindication. Believe me, I didn't feel smug about it. I just had an overwhelming, heartbreaking sense of sadness that all my suspicions – my convictions – had been proved correct.

In the first forty minutes following the attack, just one paramedic was in the City Room. He was joined by two more. And that was it. Emergency Training UK was contracted to provide medical services and first aid at the venue. But many of their staff had inadequate training.

There was no one rendezvous point. Each emergency service chose its own. Astonishingly, the fire services' rendezvous point was three miles away from the arena. Police and ambulances racing to the scene were baffled to see fire crews heading away from the blast. These fire crews, watching the tragedy unfold on social media and news websites, had been desperate to attend, but had been prevented from doing so.

By 12.01 a.m. on what was then 23 May, a full ninety minutes after the blast, just two casualties had left the casualty clearing station for hospital. By the end of the second hour, it was nine casualties. It was not until 2.50 a.m. that the final casualty departed. 'To those who experienced it, this period of time will have seemed interminable,' Sir John concluded.

It was.

The report revealed that Greater Manchester Police had correctly announced an 'Operation Plato', which was national guidance for the response to a continuing terror attack. It was, the report said, 'vital' that this was shared with other emergency services. It wasn't. GMP also failed to declare a major incident until 1 a.m. – two-and-a-half after the blast. During the 'golden hour' – the first sixty minutes in such an event – commanders should have been gathering information, making decisions, bringing order to inevitable chaos, containing and neutralising threats and rescuing victims as quickly as possible, Sir John said. 'For those who are critically injured, minutes or seconds can count.'

Tragically, heartbreakingly, Sir John concluded that one victim's life could have been saved with prompt treatment and care. And there was also a possibility, albeit remote, that a second victim, the youngest, could also have been saved. All of the emergency services issued apologies after the publication of the report.

The new chief constable for the GMP admitted that the force's failings in their response to the atrocity had 'contributed to the loss of life' and offered his unreserved apology. The chief fire officer for Greater Manchester Fire and Rescue Service also offered his 'wholehearted' apology and admitted that the force's response on the night was 'wholly inadequate' and 'totally ineffective'. 'We let the families and the public down in their time of need and for that I am truly sorry,' he said. 'I know that no apology will take away the pain and suffering of the families who lost loved ones and of the survivors. But I want them to know that I fully accept the inquiry's criticisms of our service and I accept the recommendations in full.'

The chief executive of the North West Ambulance Service admitted the force made several failings in their response to the attack. He said, 'We accept that more of our staff should have been deployed into the City Room to help triage patients and manage their evacuation. What also produces deep regret is that our ability to work together as blue-light partners fell well short of the standards we all expected. The principles of multi-agency working are incredibly important to the way we deal with major incidents. It should never have broken down so quickly and so drastically.'

Those words were all that the survivors and families of those caught up in the attack had ever wanted to hear.

In the third and final report, published in March 2023, Sir John revealed that two pieces of information about Abedi could have led to him being arrested when he returned to the UK from Libya, but they had not been passed to police by MI5. The head of MI5 released a statement saying he was 'profoundly sorry'.

Finally, after six years, the truth about what had happened that night had finally been revealed and the vilification on social media finally ceased – in one corner, at least.

The conspiracists were still at it. Over the years, I've heard various outlandish theories – that Elvis was alive and well; that the moon landings had been faked. But it was something else to hear that Eve and I had been accused of faking our own injuries and that the Manchester Arena bombing itself had been staged.

It first came to light around the first anniversary of the bombing when Lee Freeman, who had done the Great Manchester Run, was accompanying me to media interviews. On the journey home, scrolling through his social media accounts, he exclaimed, 'Bloody hell – look at this.' Glancing at his screen, I frowned, then laughed in disbelief. I looked back at Lee. Was this a joke? According to a YouTuber, the arena bombing had never happened. It was a carefully orchestrated exercise carried out by the government to enable them to introduce more stringent restrictions of public rights.

According to them, all of the 'survivors' – including Eve and me – and deceased victims had been actors, paid handsomely for our services. Now, I'm from the old school – sticks and stones may break my bones but words can never hurt me. I was far too busy with work and campaigning to give this another thought. I rolled my eyes, scoffed at the utter ridiculousness and put it out of my head. Comments continued to appear on social media, particularly whenever I spoke about my treatment with Ken and dreams of walking again. 'Miraculous recovery, eh?' some would say, snidely. My response was to delete, block and move on.

Then in the summer of 2021, Sarah rang me. One of the trolls had moved offline. 'He's boasted on the internet how he set up a camera outside our house to film Eve,' she sighed. 'He wanted to see if she really was in a wheelchair.'

I listened in sheer disbelief. A cold, hard, fury welled inside me. He's done *what?!* With trembling hands, I did some googling. Sure enough, there he was, on camera, demonstrating how and why he was using surveillance tactics to video our daughter. This man, Richard D. Hall, had been intrigued by the lack of information about Eve. There was one simple reason. In those early, awful, days after the bombing, when both Eve and I were fighting for our lives, Sarah naturally wanted to shield her from media attention. When I was well enough to be involved in our daughter's life, I agreed one hundred per cent.

Eve was just fourteen years old at the time, remember. A child. She'd suffered horrific, life-changing, injuries. As I moved on with my recovery, I was happy to give interviews and take part in documentaries. It was an opportunity to thank the people who needed thanking and expose what had gone wrong on the night. However, Sarah and I agreed that Eve should be spared attention. In many stories, I didn't even refer to my daughter by her name. I asked reporters not to include details in articles. 'She'll tell her own story once she's ready to,' I said.

Journalists understood and respected our decision. Apart from the photo of Eve and I at dinner on the night of the concert, very little was published. Yet Hall had seized upon this as proof that we were involved in a conspiracy around the Arena bombing. 'The vast majority of "victims" [yes, he used inverted commas around the word] have had considerable media coverage, so I wonder why Eve has had none?' he asked. 'Is there something about Eve that must be kept out of public view? This made me wonder whether Eve was really injured.'

Matter-of-factly, he explained how he had tracked Sarah on social media and found where she lived. He knocked on the door but, thank heavens, there was no answer. 'I left a camera running and after a few hours I returned. While I was away, three people came out of the house. Sarah, a carer and a girl in a wheelchair.' Even then, he said there was no evidence that any injury was a result of the attack.

To summarise, this is what Hall believes happened: the 2017 Manchester Arena bombing was a well-organised and well-planned fake terrorist incident involving over a hundred enlisted participants/actors. On the morning of 22 May, the actors playing the 'deceased victims' and others had all turned up to the City Room and lain down on the floor for photographs to be taken.

That evening, we'd turned up with our fake injury kits and got into position. At 10.31 p.m. an actor playing Abedi (an MI6 asset, no less) ran in to the City Room, dropped a bag containing a pyrotechnic or firework device and ran out to a getaway car. The device made a loud bang, gave off a bright flash and produced smoke. 'The actors immediately played their roles screaming and pretending to be injured,' said Hall.

Afterwards, we all gave carefully rehearsed answers in interviews. Of the deceased, most are alive and well, living new lives abroad. Hall says I'm more convincing in interviews than some of the other 'participants'. Apparently, this is due to my acting experience. I once appeared on *The Bill*, apparently, which is news to me.

I was still reeling when I was contacted by the BBC's disinformation and social media correspondent Marianna Spring. She was making a series of podcasts for BBC Radio 4 (which are still on BBC Sounds) and a *Panorama* documentary, investigating these 'disaster trolls'. Would I like to take part? Absolutely. Marianna explains in the podcasts that she'd never heard of Hall before starting her investigations. But while interviewing victims of trolling – both involved in the Arena attack and elsewhere – his name came up time and time again. 'His videos had accumulated millions of views, several dedicated to discussing what he called "fabricated terror", suggesting attacks were actually hoaxes or carried out by sinister state actors,' she said.

Through Marianna, I learned more about him and how he'd targeted my daughter – along with countless other survivors. Hall had shown viewers the surveillance device he would use to spy on Eve. It was a camera, disguised by leaves on a stick. He'd placed it inside a plant pot or, as he later claimed, running in a vehicle parked in a public place. He told viewers, 'I've got to review the footage and see who comes out of the house. It'll be interesting to see if the daughter is in that footage.' I was shaking with anger. 'The daughter'. That's how he referred to my beautiful, brave Eve.

Marianna reported on her programme, 'It was this convergence of the hatred and conspiracies online and the way it spilled into the real world, that also struck Martin hardest. He was concerned for himself, yes, but mostly he was worried about Eve, her safety, and then other survivors too, including those who lost loved ones. Hall had suggested that those who were killed in the attack are really alive and living abroad. Not only this, but he appeared to be making money from these conspiracies. He was selling books and DVDs outlining his theories at a market stall in Wales, as well as speaking at events and posting videos online.'

He had more than sixteen million views and 80,000 subscribers on YouTube. That's a lot of people being sucked into this nonsense. In my view, the people who buy into this are just as bad, just as guilty, as their interest is encouraging these outlandish theories. He's also written a book, in which he said, 'More evidence is needed to establish when, where and how the injuries were obtained. Such evidence might transpire as a result of further investigation of the participants.'

He wasn't stopping. What would he do next? And would his followers also be tempted to join in and carry out their own 'research'? In the *Panorama* documentary, Marianna tracked Hall down to his market stall in Wales, but he didn't want to talk. Bravely, she persisted. 'I just want to ask... you're selling books here. You've got your DVD, you're profiting from the worst day of these people's lives: do you realise that? How does that make you feel?' Richard said that all the answers were in his book. She said, 'I have read your book and in there there are claims about the victims that are contrary to the evidence.'

Hall wasn't backing down. 'Well, you're wrong, actually, but I don't wish to discuss it any further because I don't believe you will represent me correctly, OK?' He picked up a camcorder and began to film her.

The *Panorama* programme, which was screened in October 2022, triggered a huge reaction. I was invited on to TV to discuss it and I have to admit I was worried about a backlash. As I told Marianna for her final podcast: 'I was expecting a lot of trolling and a lot of bad comments. And literally, I didn't get one. And everything was so positive. I had MPs getting in touch with me. Obviously, a lot of my friends were upset that I'd not said anything. But I explained that's how worried I was about it.'

The publicity led to action. Hall's YouTube channels and market stall were closed down. Good.

Through the podcasts and documentary, I'd learned more about how conspiracy theories had originated in the USA. One notorious theorist, Alex Jones, had claimed on his channel that the Sandy Hook school shooting in 2012 was a hoax. In the attack, twenty-six people were murdered by one man, twenty of them children under ten. Appalled families of victims united and successfully sued Jones for defamation. He was ordered to pay them $1.5 billion in damages. But the most rewarding result was when he was forced, in court, to admit the shooting really had happened.

My brilliant legal team at Hudgell Solicitors agreed we should also take legal action. They sent Hall an initial letter, but he refused to back down and continued to sell his book and videos online. As a result of Marianna's coverage, other survivors from the arena came forward and we joined forces. In April 2023, Hudgell issued proceedings in the high court. Eve and I would be seeking an injunction to prevent Hall making similar allegations in future and suing him for defamation and harassment. It was a landmark legal action – the first of its kind in the UK.

My solicitor Neil Hudgell said, 'A number of our clients, including Martin Hibbert, have instructed us to issue proceedings against a named individual for defamation and harassment, including a claim in damages as well as for restraining injunctions. These relate to outlandish claims following the Manchester Arena atrocity that our clients are not genuine and did not suffer the life-changing injuries they did. Several of our clients have had this man on their doorstep, taking photographs, invading their privacy in the most intrusive way. Martin and others are determined to stop this individual from continuing with his repugnant behaviour.'

In the final podcast episode, bringing listeners up to date, I told Marianna, 'I'm not having people like Richard bullying people – people who can't stand up for themselves. People who don't have a voice. Well, I'm the voice. I'm the person that's going to take care of this and I'm the person that's going to change it so people like Richard can't make a living from our misery and our suffering. I'm always for freedom of speech. But he crossed the line. And when you cross the line, you always end up paying the piper. He will get what's coming.'

Part of me is saddened that it's come to this. Years ago, people like Richard D. Hall would have spouted their nonsense while standing on a soapbox at a street corner. Few would have stopped and listened. But in the age of the internet there are too many people living online, being sucked in.

Alarmingly, and as we've discovered from recent inquiries, the people we have traditionally relied upon to tell the truth – the police, the authorities, the government, aren't doing it. As a result, people are looking elsewhere for answers. Which is where people like Richard D. Hall come in: not for much longer, hopefully.

At a hearing at the high court in January 2024, we applied for a 'summary judgement' – a procedure to decide parts of the case without the need for a trial.

Hall, representing himself, was flanked by about fifty supporters, as he repeated his ridiculous claims. Incredulously, I'd had to provide receipts for the concert tickets, medical reports from my consultant and Eve's GP and witness statements from myself, Eve and her mum, Sarah. All to prove that we were there on the night and injured in the explosion.

Thankfully, Judge Richard Davison ruled in our favour. In his decision released in February he rejected Hall's theory that the Manchester bombing was an operation staged by government agencies in which no one was genuinely killed or injured as 'absurd and fantastical'.

He dismissed as 'preposterous and untenable' the claim that Eve and I received our injuries prior to the concert and were 'recruited but did not attend the concert'. And he added it was 'fanciful' to propose that Salman Abedi did not die – and still 'more fanciful' to propose that he escaped, was apprehended and then 'cleared' as a spy.

In a nutshell, Hall can no longer defend his poisonous claims and we will shortly commence proceedings on the grounds of harassment, misuse of private information and data protection breaches. Hopefully, by the summer of 2024, the case will have concluded completely.

Manchester's mayor Andy Burnham has since reached out to discuss campaigning for a new law to better protect survivors of tragedies from harassment and conspiracy theories. 'It is always difficult to change the law, and it doesn't happen overnight,' Mr Burnham said in interviews. 'But most people will see the case for this because of the appalling nature of targeting people in this way.'

I live in hope that before too long, it will be a criminal offence for people like Richard D. Hall to make money from conspiracy theories, especially in relation to terrorist attacks or atrocities. The day Eve's Law is added to the statute books will be one of the proudest moments of my life.

19

Dream Believe Achieve

I'll start this final chapter with Eve.

My brave, beautiful, strong, resilient, daughter celebrated her twenty-first birthday in October 2023. We went to TGI Friday's – her favourite restaurant – and had silver balloons festooned around her table.

My girl continues to defy medics with her remarkable recovery. She's believed to be the only person in the world to have survived such a severe brain injury. I understand a medical paper has been written to offer guidance to any doctors encountering such a wound in future. I'm more convinced than ever, now, that we were meant to survive that attack. Our lives didn't end, they just changed. Eve and I are living, breathing, medical miracles.

Yes, she will need 24/7 care for life. And it's unlikely she will ever marry or have children. Occasionally, I feel a pang, and sense of loss, for what she has missed out on and will continue to miss out on. All her peers are now driving, graduating, travelling around the world, embarking on dream jobs… It's unlikely she'll be able to do many of those things. But I pull myself back to the here and now and appreciate what I have. She's here with us. She's happy. I can hold her, hug her, talk with her, laugh with her. She's walking, talking, sending texts. They're the things we celebrate.

She's had such an impact on the wonderful people who cared for her in hospital. At some of my local speeches I've met some of the nurses who looked after her. 'How is she doing?' they ask. 'Tell her we're always thinking about her.'

We'll continue to shield her from media spotlights (and conspiracy theorists). When she's ready, Eve will tell her own story. And it will trump anything I've done!

Our Kilimanjaro climb continues to have such an impact – not only in raising essential funds but in showing others with an SCI or in a wheelchair what they can achieve with the right team and support. I was the second paraplegic in the world to reach the summit. The words roll off my tongue now, in interviews, but that sense of awe and achievement for what we did, still gives me shivers. And it's lovely to know it's giving others with spinal cord injuries hope and inspiration.

Messages come from all over the world. I was recently contacted by a man in the USA who'd been hit by a truck while out cycling. He'd been sat in a spinal rehabilitation unit, thinking his life was over. 'But I've just seen you do Kilimanjaro!' he said. Over a Zoom chat, I gave him Ken's details in Australia and advice on the best sort of wheelchair to get him out and about. And that... *that*, is what keeps me going. After a motivational speech at the Reebok Stadium, Bolton, a woman said, 'My son adores you. He's not spinal-cord injured but he's in a wheelchair and says you inspire him to live life to the full. It's not just people with an SCI you're helping but everyone in wheelchairs.' Comments like that make my day.

The climb has also meant we're spreading awareness of the help and support that is out there. Take the story of Pete Watts, for instance. Pete had lived an active life, served in the forces and was a keen mountain biker. In 2019, he bent over to pick up his shoes and ruptured a disc in the base of his spine. He underwent emergency surgery but was left with permanent nerve damage. Pete had cauda equina syndrome – a rare condition where a bundle of nerves at the base of the spine become compressed.

Let me say that again… he *bent over to pick up his shoes*. And he suffered a spinal cord injury. It can happen to anyone. And it does. Seven people a day. Every single day.

'I felt I'd lost me – they were dark days,' Pete said in an interview with *BBC Breakfast*. 'I was scrolling through my phone looking for anything that would give me hope. And there was this guy who was about to take a wheelchair up Kilimanjaro.'

Spurred on, Pete forced himself out for walks. Messages struggle to reach his legs from his brain so there are times he has to remind himself 'left leg forward, right leg forward' and uneven ground is particularly challenging. But he progressed from walking to the end of the street to walks in the park. He got in touch with the SIA and received the help he needed.

To celebrate his new, positive attitude, he's had smiley faces tattooed on each of his toes and a motto 'It's all about life!' etched along the side of his foot. Even more brilliantly, Pete has gone on to become a trustee at the SIA and now reaches out to others with SCIs. He's since climbed Snowdon, walked a marathon and completed a Superhero Tri, a triathlon for people with disabilities. That's exactly the sort of result I'd hoped for when I set out on this journey. We're not only receiving hope and encouragement but passing on the baton. However, if he hadn't learned about the SIA, found hope, where would he be?

Gary Dawson puts it so well when he says, 'Imagine a couple discovering they're pregnant – then being told by their GP, "You're on your own now. We can't do any scans or monitoring and you're going to have to deliver the baby at home, yourselves. OK?" It's unthinkable, isn't it? But that's the reality for too many people diagnosed with a spinal cord injury. You're given your wheelchair and it's a case of, "Off you go. Good luck".'

Well, sorry, but that's not good enough. It doesn't happen to patients with cancer, heart disease and diabetes. *BBC Breakfast* presenter Charlie Stayt says 'It's not good enough' has become my angry catchphrase. My dream is to use it less and less since being able to bring my fight to Westminster.

It all started when I was interviewed by Dan Walker on *BBC Breakfast*. We became friends and I was delighted, honoured and a bit stunned when he wanted to include a chapter about me in his book *Standing on their Shoulders*, about ordinary heroes. Some of the things I said – crying in the shower but living every day to the full otherwise the terrorists have won – must have resonated with him as he's spoken about me on TV quite a few times and is always championing my campaign.

While interviewing Tom Pursglove, then Minister for Disabled People, Health and Work, live on Channel 5, just before Christmas 2022, Dan brought me into the conversation. 'I've been spending a lot of time with Martin Hibbert. He said it's not the injury that makes him feel disabled but people's attitudes to him. What can we do about that?'

When Tom Pursglove replied, 'We need to talk more about that,' Dan was in there like lightning.

'He *is* talking about it,' he said. 'He regularly goes into a shop and is told, "The menswear is on the first floor and there's no lift." He goes into work and he can't get his wheelchair to fit into the lift or under the desk.'

Tom agreed that a social model of disability is about 'lowering, getting rid of, and overcoming, barriers and those very difficulties. That is a mission that I am determined to help progress in this role, looking at what specific thing we can do to try and improve that. And Martin's exactly the sort of person I'd be keen to talk to.'

Dan rang me after the show with the minister and said, 'I don't know if I've done the right thing but I've given Tom Pursglove your details.'

I was invited to the Department for Work and Pensions office in January 2023 for a meeting. Bolshy to the last, I started with, 'Today is not a day trip for me to London so you can say you've met someone in a wheelchair. I'd like you to come to the charity HQ in Milton Keynes. I'd like you in the trenches, hearing the stories we hear every day... the challenges people face every day, and the staff dealing with them.'

And to his credit, he paid a visit to the SIA headquarters two months later. He spent three hours meeting everyone and hearing about all the wonderful work the staff do. Then he told us he was going to put in place a system for ensuring that everyone with an SCI gets an automatic referral to the SIA so they can lead an active and fulfilled life. What Macmillan is to cancer patients we'd like to become the equivalent for patients with SCIs.

And that was just the start. Tom Pursglove also asked me to be part of his disability perception team and I've attended meetings with ministers. This campaign has snowballed. I grab any opportunity to fly the flag for spinal cord injuries. One highlight was Aston Martin inviting me to Silverstone to take part in a round table discussion on inclusivity and diversity. They said my Kilimanjaro climb perfectly epitomised their own 'We climb together' philosophy, a relentless drive to overcome the odds time and time again, to keep going, to keep improving, to keep climbing.

I couldn't have put it better myself. Gabby and I were like children in a sweetshop on a tour around all these gleaming motors. But the message was serious. Why shouldn't people in wheelchairs attend sporting events, shop in stores they've always loved, eat at their favourite restaurants, have stress-free journeys?

I was delighted to support TV presenter and disabilities advocate Sophie Morgan, who was left paralysed from the waist down after a car crash, aged eighteen, as she launched her Rights on Flights campaign. She was spurred into action when her wheelchair was left damaged on not one but two flights. Imagine getting off a flight only to find that the airline has lost your shoes. All of them. And there is no way of getting replacements. Now multiply that feeling of frustration, helplessness and upset by a hundred.

New research by the charity Scope, a campaign partner, shows that one in ten passengers experience negative attitudes from either airline staff or other customers; while one in fourteen are left stranded on planes without assistance after take-off or landing and have had equipment lost or damaged. As Sophie says, 'Society can no longer accept the disregard with which some disabled travellers are being treated when they fly. I've been ignored, left on planes and had expensive wheelchairs damaged. What me and my team are working on is for disabled passengers to have the same experience as other passengers. It's time to have a stronger, passenger-centric legislation so that airlines and airports can do their job better and be really held to account if they don't provide assistance to disabled people or damage equipment.'

Too right. This legislation can't come soon enough. And it should spread beyond airlines. I've taken trains where I've been unable to reach my seat let alone get into it. I've been left in my wheelchair, blocking the aisle, clinging onto a table with my fingertips for the entire journey! When booking hotels and holidays we have to ask for photos and measurements to ensure my wheelchair can actually get into the bathroom.

I haven't done any of this for accolades and awards and it's always a shock when they come along. Taking pride of place on my mantlepiece is my Points of Light award from former prime minister Boris Johnson in October 2022. The message on it is lovely. It says, 'Thank you, on behalf of everyone in the UK for what you are doing. You're inspiring not just disabled people but able-bodied people as well.' And that's really important. Because when it comes to changing perception on disability, everybody's involved.

While Chris was in Ireland, climbing yet more mountains for his son Cian's #My19 effort, the family spotted a wheelchair-friendly picnic table with a section cut away to provide access. Quick as a flash his youngest boy, Ronan, said, 'Oh look, Daddy, that's where Martin would sit if he came on a picnic with us.' And there you have it. Ronan was only four but he was already noticing inclusive features for wheelchair users. And, hopefully he will start to call out non-inclusive features as well. These children are our future MPs, ministers, lawyers, CEOs, architects. Wouldn't it be wonderful if it became second nature to them to question why awkward steps and inaccessible levels are included in building designs. Or why menswear/ladieswear/childrenswear is always on the first floor or basement in every single shop branch across the UK.

In autumn 2022, you could have knocked me down with a feather when I received a Pride of Britain regional fundraiser of the year award – live on *Granada Reports*. Presenter Zoe Muldoon surprised me at King's Cross Station café while I was waiting for a train home. It's a lovely, circular glass plaque with the words '*Daily Mirror* Pride of Britain, ITV Granada, Fundraiser Award 2022'. I couldn't take my eyes off it. Arriving home, I held it out to Gabby, who promptly burst into tears.

Attending the Pride of Britain Awards ceremony a few weeks later felt surreal. I couldn't stop thinking about my mum. She'd loved the awards and tuned in, hankies at the ready, every year. She'd have been beside herself to know I was nominated for an award. I had my photo taken with dancers from *Strictly*... (Dianne, Amy and Giovanni), Jason Fox, former UK Special Forces soldier, Royal Marine Commando and the television adventurer from *SAS: Who Dares Wins* – who is one of my heroes – and veteran boxer Frank Bruno.

Wheeling myself to the table, I passed presenter Clare Balding, who beamed as she told me, 'Ooh, you look very dapper.' *Clare Balding just complimented me!*

Gabby and I were situated quite near the walkway and we got to see all the amazing winners collect their awards. Emotions were running at full pelt – confirming, once again, how we are all climbing a mountain in some way, shape or form.

And just before I finished writing this book, I was named one of the top ten most influential disabled people on the Shaw Trust

Disability Power 100 list of 2023 – scooping the award for best community advocate – raising awareness of disability and the barriers that we face on a daily basis.

To be honest, the awards do trigger imposter syndrome. I'm just Martin from Bolton who used to nick sweets from the corner shop! But they make me proud and I know they're making Mum proud too. They're also a recognition and acknowledgement of the wonderful care I've received from so many people since the bombing. The doctors and nurses who leaped out of bed in the middle of the night to save my life. The physiotherapists who helped to fix me. They perform heroic acts day-in, day-out. Without them I simply wouldn't be here. So, I dedicate each and every award to them.

What Salman Abedi and his brother did that night was pure evil. But goodness will always prevail. I see it every single day, from the taxi driver who insists the fare is 'on him' to the random shopper in the Arndale shopping centre who says, 'Thank you for doing what you're doing. I was there that night with my own daughter...'

Then there are the wonderful friendships that I've made. I've been blessed to always have people like Karl and Steve in my life, but in the last six years my close friendship groups have swelled. Gabby pointed out that a lot of the people we spend time with now are those we've met as a result of the bombing. Yes, it was the worst night ever. But it's also introduced us to people who enrich our lives in so many ways.

There are those who were caught up on the night, like Andrea, Rob, other survivors and bereaved families; the angels who saved my life – like Mr Saxena, Paul Harvey the paramedic, Stuart Wildman my nurse and Caroline my physio. And it's not just them – but their families too. Chris, his wife and Lego-mad boys came to stay last summer, assembling my Old Trafford Lego kit in the process. I also had the honour of driving Paul's daughter, Scarlett, to her school prom. 'But Martin,' she said, gesturing to her pale blue dress. 'I'm going to get glitter all over the back seat.'

I rolled my eyes. 'Just get in!' I laughed.

She told me that arriving in a freshly valeted, dark Range Rover with a United number plate was the talk of the prom. I couldn't have been prouder. Eve had missed her own prom, her exams, her leaving assembly. That entire chapter was torn out of her life. So to play a part in another special teenager's rite of passage was truly an honour.

And then there's the brotherhood formed from climbing Kilimanjaro. The legal teams who have helped so much with our quest for justice. The journalists who enable me to keep shouting…

Almost seven years on from the atrocity, Manchester now has a living memorial garden, the Glade of Light. At the heart of the memorial is a white, marble 'halo' ring with the names of the twenty-two victims set in bronze. Personalised memory capsules, filled with precious items to commemorate the lost loved ones, are embedded within the stone. They will be there for eternity. Never forgotten.

It was an honour to be invited to the official dedication by the Duke and Duchess of Cambridge (now the Prince and Princess of Wales) on the fifth anniversary. The inscription includes the words: 'On 22 May 2017, twenty-two people – concert-goers and their loved ones waiting for them at Manchester Arena – had their lives taken in a terrorist atrocity. Many others sustained physical or mental injuries, some life-changing. The Glade of Light has been created as a memorial garden. It's a place to reflect, to remember and a lasting testament to love. We will never forget.'

Such beautiful words…

This year, I'm planning another visit to Australia to continue my NeuroPhysics Therapy journey with Ken Ware, which was put on ice during the pandemic. Ken has been instrumental in giving me the confidence and ability to forge my new, post-atrocity life. People always comment on my upright posture and core strength. And that's all down to his magic. My ambition is to bring his expertise to this country with a specialist NPT centre in Manchester. I won't rest until it's done. No one should have to travel ten thousand miles for such brilliant treatment.

And talking of brilliant treatment, the future has never looked brighter for patients with SCIs. Scientists are continually making huge advances with electrode devices and implants. The Frank Williams Academy – an initiative between the SIA and Williams Racing – has been founded to improve the lives of people with SCIs. And the work by the late Christopher Reeve – a real-life Superman – to find a cure for spinal cord injury is being continued by his foundation and his children. I'm convinced that bright days are just around the corner.

You might like to know that the very wheelchair that took me up Kilimanjaro is still working its magic. It was the top prize in an Everyday Mountains competition run by the SIA and was awarded to Emma Cawood from Leeds, who was paralysed at the start of lockdown. She told a journalist, 'I haven't been able to go out with my family on dog walks. I haven't been able to go out with my son who loves to go mountain biking. I have had this dream for a while now to go up Snowdon and it wouldn't be possible in my current chair. This is going to be life-changing. My world is just going to open up.' I confess to having something in my eye when hearing those words.

For now, I'm continuing to shout about everything from depression (let's talk about it) to greater awareness of sepsis (I've succumbed seven times now) and, of course, spinal cord injuries. I like to think, in some small way, I'm making a difference – and encouraging others to join me.

One of my recent inspirational talks was in Chicago to two thousand people. The organisers asked me to choose some uplifting music to wheel myself on stage to. I thought and thought. I racked my brains. I lay awake at night. And then, I finally confessed I couldn't do it. 'I'm going to look like David Brent coming out on stage!' I argued, picturing Ricky Gervais's deluded middle-manager from *The Office*. Instead, I suggested news footage unfolding from the night of the atrocity. The result? Ninety seconds of dramatic newsfeeds, breaking news reports, blue, flashing lights surrounding the arena, the wounded being helped, the tributes at St Ann's Square. As the film finishes, the lights come on and the audience knows exactly why I'm there, on stage, in a wheelchair. I use it for all my talks now and finish with the Tony Walsh poem (which still brings me to tears every time I hear it).

Losing my dear friend, Mike, my surrogate dad, on 23 September 2020 – Mum's birthday – was a true reminder of just how short and precious life is. It's the same with that now infamous picture of me and Eve, captured just a few hours before the explosion. It will always be a poignant reminder of what life might have been. However, I would also hope it can serve as a reminder of how life should be lived, no matter what circumstances befall us.

People joke that the Hibberts have dragon's blood running through their veins. My grandparents, who toiled in the cotton mills, instilled in me a sense of working hard and getting on with it. Their belief was there will always be times when life doesn't seem bearable – but you just dust yourself down and get on with it. These are the cards you've been dealt. You either sit in the corner and mope or you get up and make the best of it.

And that is what Eve and I are both doing. We were privileged in being the closest people to the bombing to survive. So many around us died that night.

Shortly after the bombing, I remember saying in interviews, 'We really shouldn't be here. I'm not religious but I truly believe we were saved for a reason.'

It's taken seven years, but finally, I understand the answer – to shout my 'Dream Believe Achieve' mantra from the rafters.

As the brilliant Tony Walsh says in his poem Everyday Mountains:

'And Martin? He's just starting
… and he's never gonna stop!'

THE END…

Acknowledgements

When it was first suggested I write a book, I was stunned. 'Give over,' was my initial response.

And then I thought of me mum. She'd have been so bloody proud – hovering around bookshelves, pointing out the cover and delightedly telling passersby, 'That's our Martin, that is/that's Martin, my boy.'

So Mum... this is for you. Thank you for your love, guidance and patience – all qualities that have made me the man I am today. I miss you so much and I hope I make you proud every day.

There are so many people I need to thank and acknowledge.

My beautiful daughter Eve, the most precious person in my life and my absolute world. Your smile is all I need to remind me how lucky I am to be your dad. I know you will inspire the world when you are ready.

My soulmate Gabby... my life, my love, my heart, my everything. Always. Thank you for always being by my side. I love you so much.

Danny and Andy; the best brothers anyone could ever wish for. It's true what they say... There is no love like the love for a brother and there is no love like the love from a brother.

Granddad Bob – my role model and real life hero. You taught me so much and I am forever grateful.

Patricia, Peter and Pam - thank you for the love, help and support that you continually give to me, Gabby and Alfie.

Sarah, thank you for everything you do for Eve and making sure she is safe and happy. You're an amazing mum.

Steve, some people make such a profound impact that you can barely remember what life was like without them. Thank you for your love and support and always being there.

Karl, there are friends, there is family and then there are friends that become family. You are the person I look up to and always want to make proud. Thank you for your love, friendship and keeping my feet on the ground.

Paul, thank you for what you did that night. You are a friend for life and I'm forever in your debt.

Ankur, a true friend and brilliant doctor. You are the reason I am still alive and able to climb mountains. Thank you for saving my life and being a big part of it.

Stuart, what a journey we've been on together since I first arrived battered and broken on your ward. I am so grateful to have you in my life and so proud to be able to call you my friend.

Caroline, there are certain people who make the world a better place just by being in it. You are one of those people. I love you, my friend.

To Chris, Rob and the entire team who helped me reach the Top of the World. And to all the wonderful friends and colleagues who have been there for me both before the atrocity and afterwards. I'm blessed to be surrounded by you. Apologies if I haven't mentioned you by name but you know who you are.

To Mandy, my second mum and a beautiful angel. I will never forget the love, care and support you gave me. I am blessed to have you in my life. And Mike, my best man and father figure. You are loved and missed.

Salford Royal Infirmary: 'For he who has health has hope and he who has hope has everything.' To all the amazing people who work there. Thank you for all you have done and continue to do for me and my family. And to every medic who has looked after me so well during my many visits. You really are life's true angels.

Fiona, just think we were complete strangers until a few years ago and now you know everything about me! The good and the bad! Thank you for your help and guidance in writing this book. It's been a journey, but one I will be forever grateful for. I hope you are as proud of the book as I am.

To Gary and everyone at the Spinal Injuries Association. Thank you for the difference you have made to my life and others with spinal cord injuries.

To Ken and Nickie at NeuroPhysics Therapy in Australia. Thank you for believing in me and enabling me to find, deep inside, the best version of myself. You are true miracle workers.

Richard, my wonderful chiropodist (now looking after Eve's feet) and gym buddy. You have made such a difference to my life in so many ways.

To the brilliant Tony Walsh. Thank you for your incredibly moving words and for allowing me the honour of including them in this book.

Mike, Lianne and Mike's mum Wendy at Digs4Dogs. It's not just Alfie who loves you. You are the most wonderful people and we honestly don't know how we'd have managed without you all these years.

To the wonderful legal teams at Hudgell and Irwin Mitchell – and Andrea. Thank you for ensuring that all those who were affected that night were listened to.

To Duncan Proudfoot at Ad Lib Publishers, and Robert Smith, my literary agent, thank you for your belief and investment in my story.

And thanks also to Layla Jenkins at Room54, BBC Radio Manchester, *BBC Breakfast*, *Good Morning Britain* and all the journalists who have given me a voice over the last six years.

Piers Morgan – for keeping me going during many dark early mornings in hospital; Chris Hemsworth – a god both on the screen and in real life and Dan Walker for all you have done and continue to do.

And a final, heartfelt, thank you to every single person who has generously supported my fundraising. You have made such a difference to so many lives.